Avoiding the First Cause of Death

Avoiding the First Cause of Death

Can We Live
Longer than 120 years?

2nd edition with guidelines

Wulf Dröge

iUniverse, Inc.
New York   Bloomington

Avoiding the First Cause of Death
Can We Live Longer than 120 years?

The information, ideas, and suggestions in this book are not intended
as a substitute for professional medical advice. Before following any
suggestions contained in this book, you should consult your personal
physician. Neither the author nor the publisher shall be liable or
responsible for any loss or damage allegedly arising as a consequence of
your use or application of any information or suggestions in this book.

iUniverse books may be ordered through booksellers or by contacting:
iUniverse
1663 Liberty Drive
Bloomington, IN 47403
www.iuniverse.com
1-800-Authors (1-800-288-4677)

Because of the dynamic nature of the Internet, any Web addresses or links contained in
this book may have changed since publication and may no longer be valid. The views
expressed in this work are solely those of the author and do not necessarily reflect the
views of the publisher, and the publisher hereby disclaims any responsibility for them.

ISBN: 978-1-4401-3949-9 (sc)
ISBN: 978-1-4401-3951-2 (hc)
ISBN: 978-1-4401-3950-5 (e-book)

Library of Congress Control Number 2009927961

Printed in the United States of America

iUniverse rev. date: 9/23/2009

Contents

Preface

Interventions that delay aging are expected to improve health and the quality of life in old age. The US National Institute on Aging's Interventions Testing Program (ITP) has recently been established to test compounds of interest for effects on aging in mice. Rapamycin was the first compound that consistently caused an increase in maximum life span in mice which started receiving this treatment at 600 days of age corresponding to 60 years in humans (Harrison et al. July 2009. *Nature* 460:392-395). As this compound inhibits the "Target Of Rapamycin" (TOR/mTOR), a key element in the insulin signaling cascade, rapamycin was expected to have similar effects as the genetic mutation of the insulin receptor analogue in the round worm *C.elegans* which was previously shown to increase the maximum life span by more than 250 percent. The subsequent discovery that the mutation of one of several genes in this signaling cascade caused a substantial but finite increase in maximum life span in several animal species suggested 1) that the maximum life span in several animal species and probably humans is limited by the first of several mechanisms of death, and 2) that humans may possibly gain a few more decades beyond 120 years by overcoming this "first cause of death".

Unfortunately, repamycin has some adverse affects that are discussed in this book and that still need to be studied in more detail. This book therefore takes a look into the underlying mechanisms and describes several natural interventions that target the same biological mechanisms as rapamycin but are not relying on pharmacological drugs. These interventions which are based on a broad range of scientific evidence are likely to decrease the rate of aging. It would be unwise to ignore the chances.

The detailed knowledge of the underlying mechanisms may also help the reader to incorporate the principles of life span extension into his or her life. As most life span extending mutations or interventions tend to enhance the "removal of cellular waste" by regulated "self-cannibalism" at the expense of protein synthesis, this book contains additional sections that may help especially the elderly to strengthen skeletal muscle protein synthesis and muscle function. Optimizing self-rejuvenation means to alternate between periods of rigorous "self-destruction" and vigorous reconstruction; but one may always keep in mind that the invisible phase of "self-destruction" and cellular "waste-removal" is the relatively more critical determinant of longevity.

WARNING: This book is medicine and not poetry. If you make up your mind and think that the quality of life during the next 50 years is important for you, then you may want to read this book. Non-specialists may want to skip over the scientific evidence when reading this book for the first time.

Anti-aging books typically promise the readers to add a couple of years to their lives by improving their lifestyles. This book is addressed to readers who are already health aficionados and who are now asking whether they could possibly live beyond the maximum human life span of about 120 years.

Introduction

Life Span Extension in Animals and the Concept
of the First Cause of Death

Those who are not succumbing to coronary heart disease, cancer, or other causes of earlier death will have the privilege to approach the maximum human life span. The longest well-documented human life span is that of Jeanne Calment of France who died in 1997 at the age of 122 years and 164 days. The period of approximately 120 years is therefore viewed as the maximum human life span. To get even close to this life span one obviously has to live a healthy life. But can one still live better than well? Can one reach beyond the maximum life span?

To address this question, one needs to ask "what is the ultimate cause of death"? This book describes a new scientific concept of the biological process of dying and presents some practical recommendations that may give complying people a few more decades to live and a better quality of life in old age. A broad range of scientific evidence suggests that the current maximum life span of man and most animals is primarily determined by a complex set of biological mechanisms that collectively form the first cause of death. First cause of death refers to the concept that there are, in addition, various other mechanisms that can also cause death but happen to be slower and may only take their toll later if the first cause of death could be eliminated.

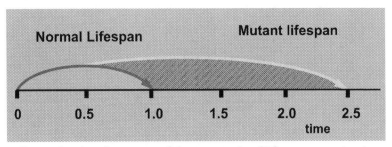

Fig. 1. Graphic illustration of the magnitude of life span extension in
longevity mutants of *C.elegans*, a roundworm. The numbers indicate
multiples of the normal life span.

The concept of the first cause of death and our knowledge about
the underlying mechanisms and its putative role in the human species
are mainly based on the discovery of certain mutants of worms, flies,
and mice, which unexpectedly showed an increase in maximum life
span by up to two-and-a-half fold (figure 1).

At least in one case, the mutation was also shown to ameliorate
certain symptoms of aging, such as the deterioration of muscle
function. As this life span extension was still limited and achieved
by mutation of a single gene, it seems reasonable to assume that one
cause of death, that is the first cause of death, had been "inactivated"
and replaced by a second one that needs more time to take its toll.

The term first cause of death should therefore be distinguished
from the major causes of death, such as cardiovascular diseases or
cancer, although these may well be mechanistically related to the
first cause of death.

In view of the available evidence the author reached the
conclusion that the process of rejuvenation depends above all on
alternating periods of rigorous self-cannibalism which removes
waste from the body, and effective reconstruction. The decline and
eventual insufficiency of the mechanism of self-cannibalism appears
to be the most critical part of the first cause of death. To ameliorate
the aging-related changes one may thoughtfully use any minute of
the day to render the periods of self-cannibalism during the night
and reconstruction during the day as effective as possible

Chapter One

The Importance of Eating Yourself

Recycling of cellular "waste" as a Critical Basis for Rejuvenation and Longevity in Animal Mutants with Extended Life Span

Detailed research on several longevity mutants of worms revealed the observed increase in maximum life span involved a biological mechanism of controlled self-destruction known as *autophagy*, literally "self-eating." A biological signal that normally adjusts this autophagic process to a relatively moderate level was inactivated in these mutants, and autophagy was accordingly increased. Work from many laboratories now collectively suggests that autophagy is an important key to the understanding of longevity.

Among other physiological functions, autophagy is responsible for the removal of cellular waste, which accumulates in cells and tissues in the course of aging in both man and animals (figure 2).

As the products of the breakdown of proteins (the free amino acids) are being used for the synthesis of new proteins, autophagy is the centerpiece of a waste recycling mechanism. Just as the constant renewal of an old city requires the continuous removal of old and rotten objects to obtain space for new and modern structures, the self-rejuvenation of higher organisms critically depends on the

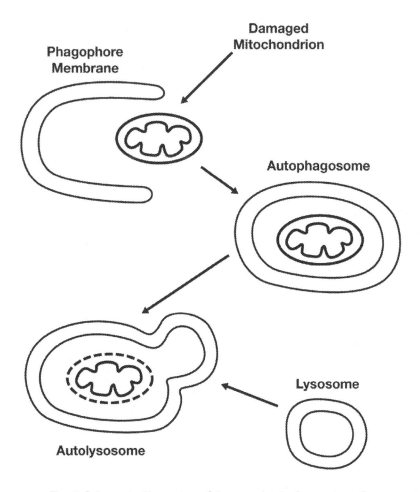

Fig. 2. Schematic illustration of the autophagic destruction of a mitochondrion. A double-layer membrane (phagophore) engulfs a damaged mitochondrion. The resulting envelope (autophagosome) subsequently fuses with another organelle (lysosome) to yield the autolysosome. The aggressive mix of lysosomal enzymes leads to the destruction of the mitochondrion.

removal of all sorts of waste that would otherwise compromise the formation of new structures. For example, it is a big challenge for the cells to get rid of damaged mitochondria, the power plants of the cells. Due to their job as an energy source of the cells, mitochondria are easily damaged. Because they are big and complex structures, damaged mitochondria are not easily broken down and removed. The mechanism of autophagy typically does this difficult and important job. Adequate autophagic waste recycling is therefore critically needed for self-rejuvenation. But, as aging cells and tissues show a conspicuous accumulation of damaged mitochondria and other forms of cellular waste in both animals and man, it is obvious that the autophagic activity becomes insufficient in old age.

Even small organisms, such as worms and flies, are complex structures, and many different vital processes can go wrong and potentially cause death. However, the spectacular increase in the life span of worms in which the autophagic activity was increased indicated the failure to ensure adequate autophagic waste recycling is simply the first failure most likely to kill or at least part of this cause of death. The following sections will present further arguments and supportive evidence to suggest this conclusion may also apply to man. There is reason to believe that the insufficient rate of autophagy in old age is an important part of the mechanism that determines the maximum life span of man and most animal species.

Signals Involved in the Regulation of "Waste Recycling" Activity

Several longevity mutants showed defects in a signaling mechanism that normally slow the rate of autophagic waste recycling. The importance of autophagy was subsequently confirmed by showing that life span extension was prevented if the mutants had, in addition to this kind of signaling defect, a second defect that impaired the autophagic process. The biological signaling mechanism responsible for the regulation of autophagy is very ancient and already found in worms as well as man. For the purpose of this book, one may simply call it the *insulin signaling mechanism* because, surprisingly, this signaling mechanism was found to be homologous (and even identical in humans) to the signaling mechanisms that control the response to insulin, the important metabolic hormone, and insulin-like growth factor I (IGF-I). Previously, insulin was mainly known for its role in diabetes and less for its role in the regulation of autophagy. For the purpose of this book, it is important to remember that the insulin signaling mechanism *inhibits* autophagy (figure 3).

In clinical medicine, the hormone insulin is widely known for its important role in glucose metabolism and body fat deposition. It is best known for its role in diabetic patients, where insufficient levels of insulin lead to abnormally high glucose levels in the blood. In addition to its role in glucose clearance from the blood, insulin also stimulates the synthesis of proteins in skeletal muscle and other tissues, provided that sufficient amounts of free amino acids are available that serve as the building blocks of proteins. Upregulation of protein synthesis involves the insulin signaling mechanism (figure 3). In humans, most of the protein synthesis happens during daytime when the consumption of proteins and carbohydrates raise blood levels of amino acids and insulin. Incidentally and through the same signaling mechanism, the increase in amino acid and insulin concentrations suppresses the autophagic waste destruction during most of the day (figure 3).

Autophagic waste destruction thus happens mainly in the fasted state, that is, during periods of starvation. In man, autophagy happens mainly at night (figure 4). In the fasted state when amino acid and insulin concentrations in the blood are low, protein synthesis is largely shut down, and autophagy is allowed to proceed. The resulting nightly autophagic protein breakdown is usually so strong that it causes skeletal muscle tissues to release substantial amounts of the resulting free amino acids into the blood. During daytime, muscle tissues typically take up amino acids from the blood to synthesize proteins. In humans, these changes between release and uptake of amino acids can easily be measured by determining the amino acid concentrations in the arteries and veins of the lower extremities.

The importance of "Waste Recycling" in times of Starvation

Whereas starvation is needed to release the brakes that control the autophagic waste destruction, autophagy ensures the survival of the organism under starving conditions by preventing a shortage in free amino acids. Simply, garbage recycling is most important when new raw materials are not available. To avoid excessive autophagic self-destruction , this process is controlled by a feedback mechanism and stops when its products, the amino acids, have reached adequate

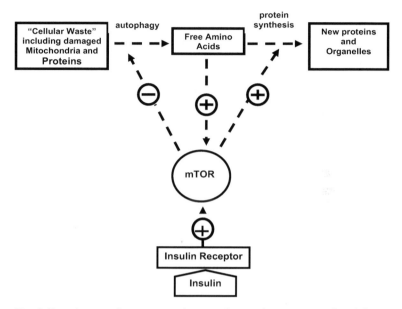

Fig. 3. Regulation of protein synthesis and autophagic protein breakdown
by the insulin receptor signaling mechanism. Autophagy converts
proteins from damaged mitochondria and other forms of cellular
waste into free amino acids. The resulting increase in free amino acid
concentrations eventually activates the signaling protein mTOR, which
then suppresses the autophagic activity. This feedback regulation plays a
key role in the maintenance of adequate free amino acid concentrations
(amino acid homeostasis) during starvation. After intake of dietary
protein and carbohydrate, the resulting increase in the plasma amino acid
and insulin concentrations activates mTOR and effectively stimulates
protein synthesis while suppressing autophagic activity.

concentrations (figure 3). In essence, this is a concentration-
dependent inhibition of autophagy by a subset of free amino acids
defined as *regulatory amino acids*. The most prominent regulatory
amino acid is leucine. Autophagy stops, and the resulting release of
free amino acids comes to an end if these amino acids reach a certain
equilibrium. Through this process, autophagy ensures the maintenance
of adequate free amino acid concentrations during nighttime and
extended periods of starvation. This process is called *amino acid
homeostasis*. It is the other vital biological function of autophagy.

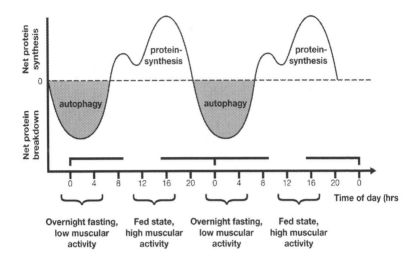

Fig. 4. Circadian variation in autophagic activity and protein synthesis. Autophagic activity is maximally expressed during periods of starvation, that is, during the night when protein synthesis is typically low. During daytime, the dietary protein/amino acid intake and high insulin levels in response to dietary carbohydrate stimulate protein synthesis and suppress the autophagic protein breakdown. Autophagic processes and their two vital functions, cellular waste removal and amino acid homeostasis, occur mainly in the fasted state during nighttime. During this period, autophagy also provides most of the cysteine that is needed for glutathione synthesis and the defense against oxidative stress. In contrast, the replacement of lost proteins and cellular constituents by novel protein synthesis happens mostly in the fed state during daytime. During this period, glutathione biosynthesis can be maintained largely by cysteine from dietary protein.

Scientific Evidence

Autophagy as a mechanism of waste removal

Autophagy is an evolutionary conserved mechanism by which cytoplasmic material is engulfed by intracellular membranes from endoplasmic reticulum, which thereby form double-layer vesicles (autophagosomes) (figure 2). These autophagosomes eventually fuse with lysosomes (370, 192). By degrading damaged organelles and long-lived proteins, autophagy plays an important role in the maintenance of cellular integrity (296, 1, 370, 192, 31, 265). The removal of mitochondria by autophagosomes is well-documented (383, 250, 236, 134, 41, 382, 110, 370, 192). As the mitochondrial permeability transition was found to initiate autophagy (110), stressed mitochondria may be a preferred target for autophagy. Autophagy also plays a major role in the turnover of cellular proteins and may be important for the catabolism of Alzheimer's precursor protein (reviewed in 84, 186, 348, 30). So it makes sense that the mechanisms that regulate the rate of autophagy also have a strong effect on the speed of aging, as illustrated by the genetic studies described previously. The impact of age on the physiological regulation of autophagic activity therefore deserves special attention.

Autophagy as the key to life span

The fact that the mutation of a single gene can result in a substantial increase in life span was first discovered in 1993 in *C. elegans*, a type of roundworm (181), which around that time had begun to establish itself in research laboratories as one of the most useful small, multicellular animals. Subsequently, a similar life span extension was also found in the common fruit fly and even mice. Surprisingly, several longevity strains of *C. elegans* and the common fruit fly were found to involve mutations in components or homologues of the insulin receptor signaling pathway (181, 100, 165, 178, 17, 189, 255). Some of these mutants showed a maximum life span two-and-a-half times greater and, in one case, even ten times greater than that of the wild type. In one study on flies, the mutation was also shown to ameliorate the functional decline (377). In both mice (219) and humans (reviewed in 364), genetic variants with reduced insulin signaling and IGF-1 signaling activity were associated with long survival, indicating similar mechanisms are limiting the life span of a broad range of species. In *C. elegans*, strong mutations in daf genes led to an abnormal development called *dauer formation* even under favorable conditions, whereas some weak mutations in the daf-2 gene that codes for the insulin receptor homologue of the worm was shown to prolong life span without significantly altering development (181).

These findings were surprising as they implicated a negative role of a well-known signaling pathway, which was previously known for its important positive role in the regulation of glucose clearance and other metabolic functions in humans. The detailed analysis showed that the insulin receptor signaling pathway downregulates the autophagic protein catabolism through the serine/threonine kinase Akt1/2 (PDB) and the target of rapamycin (TOR or mTOR in mammals) (267, 344). Mutations in this signaling pathway therefore lead to an increase in autophagic activity. That the autophagic activity is indeed required for life span extension has been shown by targeting different autophagy genes in two independent genetic studies in *C. elegans* (150, 244).

The life span extension by the daf-2 mutation in worms was shown to also require an intact daf-16 gene that codes for the transcription factor DAF-16, a homologue of the forkhead (FOXO) transcription factors that are similarly found in mammalian animals and humans (181). Like autophagy, the function of FOXO proteins is downregulated by the insulin signaling mechanism through phosphorylation by protein kinase Akt/PKB and maximally derepressed under conditions of starvation. In flies, overexpression of FOXO was shown to be sufficient for life span extension (165) and prevented the age-related decline in cardiac function (377). The mammalian FOXO-1 and FOXO-3 transcription factors were shown to induce the expression of proteins involved in both the autophagic/lysosomal pathway and the ubiquitin-proteasomal pathway of proteolysis (232, 386, 339, 304, 307). In contrast to the role of autophagy in the removal of defective organelles, the proteasomal pathway accounts for the turnover of damaged, long-lived muscular proteins that are not degraded through the autophagic/lysosomal pathway (335). In humans, variants in FOXO-1 and FOXO-3 genes segregated with survival to age eighty-five and older (reviewed in 364). FOXO was found to interact with SIRT1, the human orthologue of silent information regulator 2 (SIR2) protein deacetylase, another longevity-modulating protein (reviewed in 364).

These studies should not be interpreted to mean the derepression of autophagic activity is sufficient to increase the life span. Quite possibly, additional factors and mechanisms may be involved. But, in view of its role in the removal of aging-related cellular waste, the turnover and rejuvenation of organelles and long-lived proteins, the generation of free amino acids during fasting, and indirectly in the control of oxidative stress, autophagy appears to be a most promising target in attempts to ameliorate aging-related degenerative processes (31). Two independent studies in mice have shown that loss of autophagy in the central nervous system causes neurodegeneration and a shortened life span (147, 193). Mice genetically engineered to lack either of the autophagy genes, Atg5 or Atg7, in neuronal cells during later stages of embryogenesis develop signs of neurodegeneration and eventually show inclusion bodies akin to those seen in various human aging-related neurodegenerative disorders (147, 193).

Aging-related decline in autophagic activity

Several animal studies have shown the formation of autophagosomes decreases with age (93, 342, 347). Electron microscopic studies and measurements of the amino acid release in rats revealed the highest rates of postabsorptive (autophagic) proteolysis and the greatest sensitivity to changes in amino acid concentrations occurred at six months of age and declined thereafter (93). Another indication for an age-related decline in autophagic activity is the age-related accumulation of damaged mitochondria and other forms of biological waste in skeletal muscle fibers, neurons, and other postmitotic cells (93). It is a common finding in old age that structurally abnormal mitochondria accumulate in postmitotic cells, mitochondrial oxidative phosphorylation decreases, and mitochondrial hydrogen peroxide production increases accordingly (149, 28, 298, 259, 331). The latter indicates that at least some of the abnormal mitochondria have defective electron transport chains and produce abnormally high amounts of superoxide radicals (O_2^-), giving rise to hydrogen peroxide and other reactive oxygen species (ROS).

Superoxide radicals and other ROS induce mitochondrial DNA deletion mutants (222), which have been hypothesized to outreplicate the wild-type mitochondrial DNA genome (242). In senescent cells and tissues, ROS may also cause lipofuscin deposits (250, 236), which have been hypothesized to compromise the autophagic removal of defective mitochondria (44). Further studies linking a decrease in autophagic activity to an increase in oxidative stress are described later.

11

Note added in proof: A recent study on autophagy-defective Atg5(-/-) cells showed that these cells accumulated dysfunctional mitochondria associated with increased levels of ROS (Tal, M.C., and colleagues. 2009.Proc Natl Acad Sci USA106:2770-2775)

Role of autophagy in amino acid homeostasis

Several studies showed that the autophagic protein catabolism also plays a key role in the maintenance of adequate free amino acid concentrations under starving (postabsorptive) conditions (214, 326). By increasing the free amino acid concentration, autophagy can become essential for cell survival at times of limited amino acid availability, as most strikingly demonstrated in budding yeast (*Saccharomyces cerevisiae*) and slime mold (*Dictyostelium discoideum*) (358, 272, 192). However, as autophagy is essentially a mechanism of self-destruction, it needs to be tightly regulated. To prevent excessive and potentially harmful autocannibalism, autophagy is negatively controlled by the same signaling pathway that positively controls the rate of protein synthesis, that is, by the insulin receptor signaling cascade and its key regulator, the target of rapamycin (TOR and mTOR in mammals) (85, 104, 267). Because mTOR is activated by increasing concentrations of free amino acids and it negatively controls autophagic activity, this system provides an almost perfect autoregulatory loop that stops autophagy when free amino acid concentrations increase and reach a certain level. At this point, the system is in equilibrium (reviewed in 107) (figure 3).

In humans, the insulin- and amino acid-sensitive postabsorptive autophagic net protein catabolism in the skeletal muscle tissue can be conveniently measured by determining the amino acid exchange rate across the lower extremities. This exchange rate is the difference between the plasma amino acid concentrations in the femoral artery and the femoral vein multiplied by the blood flow (32, 343, 365). Such amino acid exchange studies have shown that peripheral tissues (mainly skeletal muscle) take up amino acids after a meal (during the postprandial state) and release amino acids in the postabsorptive (fasted) state, that is, in a state with relatively low plasma insulin and amino acid levels. The postabsorptive release of amino acids is strongly inhibited by infusion of insulin or an exogenous supply of amino acids, suggesting this process is mainly mediated by the lysosomal/autophagic mechanism of protein catabolism because autophagy is the only known proteolytic mechanism that is regulated in this way (32, 94, 131, 134, 257, 289, 343, 365).

Chapter Two

*The Effect of Aging on the Glutathione Level
and Oxidative Stress*

Additional Consequences of the Aging-related Decline in "Waste Recycling" Activity

As autophagy plays a key role in the maintainance of free amino acid levels, it is not unexpected that the age-related decline in autophagic activity is associated not only with an accumulation of cellular waste but also with a change in amino acid homeostasis. This effect has been demonstrated in humans by showing the plasma concentrations of the two amino acids, cysteine and asparagine, in the fasted state decrease with age.

The age-related decrease in the plasma cysteine concentration in the fasted state (during the night) has particularly undesirable consequences for the aging process because cysteine is needed for the synthesis of glutathione, the quantitatively most important intracellular scavenger of oxygen radicals. Glutathione is also needed for the removal of the aggressive compound hydrogen peroxide which is generated from oxygen radicals. As the plasma cysteine concentration decreases under starving conditions and in old age, so does the glutathione level. As a consequence, old age is associated with increased levels of oxygen radicals and hydrogen peroxide, which eventually lead to a condition called *oxidative stress*. Many people correctly view oxidative stress and free radicals as important causes of tissue damage and health hazards, but they associate these terms merely with the recommendation to take antioxidant vitamins that are widely popular as health supplements. This is an oversimplification, and it misses the point that glutathione is a much more important antioxidant and radical scavenger than these vitamins. Through the important role of glutathione, the widely known buzz words of *oxidative stress* and *oxygen radicals* are intimately linked to the progressive decline in autophagic waste recycling.

The concommitant decrease of both cysteine and asparagine was an important finding in this context because it showed the connection between the age-related decrease in glutathione levels and the decrease in amino acid homeostasis and autophagic acitivity. The combined evidence from different fields of research is thus leading to the paradigm that the autophagic activity decreases progressively with age and causes a shift in amino acid homeostasis and decrease in postabsorptive plasma cysteine concentration, which, in turn, causes a decrease in glutathione and corresponding increase in oxidative stress.

A Vicious Cycle that Explains the Decline in "Waste Recycling" Activity

Oxidative stress causes aberrant insulin signaling activity. The metabolic hormone insulin is best known for its role in stimulating the clearance of glucose from the blood after carbohydrate consumption. An inadequate response to insulin is one of the key problems in patients with type 2 diabetes. Could one really expect to increase the human life span by decreasing the insulin signaling activity? The answer is that one does want to have a strong insulin signal during the day in response to food consumption, but one also wants an essentially complete silence of the insulin signaling mechanism during periods of starvation to ensure maximum derepression of the autophagic activity. Ideally, the insulin signaling mechanism should operate like "a well-tuned automobile which idles quietly at the intersection but responds promptly and well when the light changes" (to use a metaphor of Weindruch and Walford from 1988). This basal insulin signaling activity under conditions of starvation needs to be decreased as much as possible to optimize the autophagic activity (figure 3).

But, even in the young and healthy organism, the basal signaling activity from the insulin receptor is never completely zero. Importantly, this signaling activity is triggered not only by insulin but also by oxygen radicals and hydrogen peroxide, even in the absence of insulin. It is well-documented that several components of the insulin signaling mechanism respond to oxygen radicals and hydrogen peroxide in such a way that, overall, the signal is enhanced. This also happens in young, healthy individuals where oxygen radicals play a role in the normal regulation of this signaling pathway. If present at appropriate concentrations, oxygen radicals and hydrogen peroxide indeed have an important positive function in the regulation of physiological signaling processes. For this purpose, almost all cells and tissues contain special enzymes that produce oxygen radicals and hydrogen peroxide at a well-regulated rate. But, under conditions of abnormally low glutathione levels, as they occur in old age, the increased levels of oxygen radicals and hydrogen peroxide disturb these regulatory processes. Among other problems, these increased levels cause an aberrant activation of the insulin signaling mechanism and compromise the silencing of the insulin signaling mechanism in the fasted state. As a consequence, the age-related increase in oxidative stress accounts partly or even completely for the decline in autophagic activity.

The physiological role of the stimulatory effect of oxygen radicals on the insulin signaling mechanism has been demonstrated in several clinical studies. Most impressively, in women, it was shown that late pregnancy is associated with an increased ability to scavenge hydrogen peroxide. This increase is quantitatively correlated with a decrease in insulin responsiveness. This effect is expected to increase the postabsorptive plasma cysteine level, thereby supporting the developing fetus and production of cysteine-rich milk proteins during lactation. In another study, insulin responsiveness under fasted conditions was shown to be decreased by cysteine supplementation. This effect is potentially useful as it reverses the aberrant stimulation of the insulin signaling activity in the fasted state. This desirable effect provides the basis for one of the interventions described in chapter five. The available information can be summarized in the following points:

- The aberrant activation of the insulin signaling mechanism under oxidative conditions inevitably affects the rate of autophagic waste destruction and indirectly impacts the maintenance of adequate plasma amino acid concentrations, including cysteine levels, under starving conditions during the night and early morning hours. Ultimately, the decrease in cysteine leads to a decrease in glutathione and increase in oxidative stress. This mechanism constitutes a vicious cycle and provides a simple explanation for the progressive age-related increase in oxidative stress as illustrated in figure 5. As the inadequate clearance of cellular waste, decreased glutathione level, and various manifestations of oxidative damage are hallmarks of old age in a broad range of species, including humans, the vicious cycle in figure 5 can be viewed as a common first cause of death. If so, life span extension may be achieved by any biochemical pathway, mutation, or intervention that effectively interacts with this cycle at any point. The existence of different types of longevity mutants (chapter three) and the life span extension by treatment with rapamycin (chapter five) support this conclusion.

- The knowledge about this cycle may lead to useful applications.

- Measuring the plasma cysteine and asparagine concentrations in the starved state may be the least invasive method to monitor at any given time the state of this vicious cycle in a given person.

Scientific Evidence

Changes in amino acid homeostasis as a cause of oxidative stress

A study of more than two hundred healthy human subjects between the third and ninth decade of life revealed a significant decrease in the postabsorptive plasma concentration of non-protein thiol and asparagine (142, 158) (figure 6). Non-protein thiol can be considered as an approximate measure of plasma cysteine because the plasma concentrations of glutathione and other low molecular weight thiol compounds are very low in comparison to the plasma cysteine

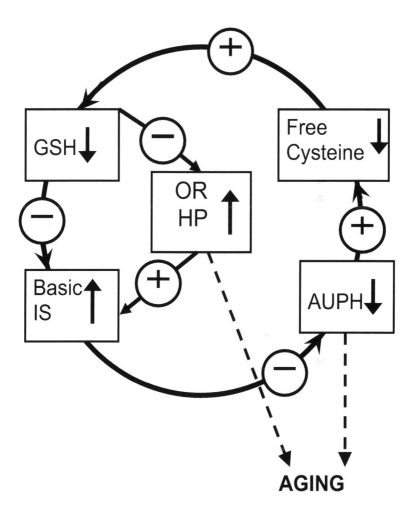

Fig. 5. A vicious cycle causing a progressive decrease in autophagic activity and an increase in oxidative stress in aging. The insulin-independent oxidative enhancement of the insulin signaling mechanism in the starved condition (basic IS) leads to a decrease in autophagic activity (AUPH) and amino acid homeostasis. The resulting decrease in the postabsorptive plasma cysteine concentration causes a decrease in intracellular glutathione (GSH) and a corresponding increase in oxygen radicals (OR) and hydrogen peroxide (HP), which ultimately leads to a further insulin-independent upregulation of the (basic) insulin signaling mechanism (107).

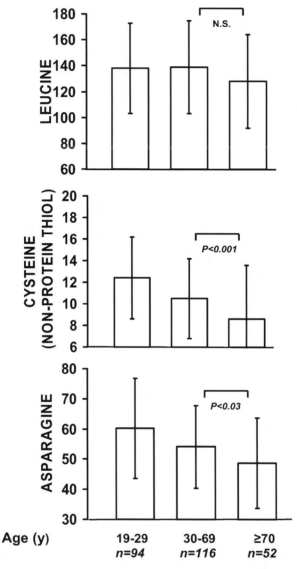

Fig. 6. Age-related changes in fasting plasma amino acid concentrations ($\mu M \pm S.D.$) A study of 262 healthy human volunteers between the second and tenth decade of life revealed a significant age-related decrease in the postabsorptive plasma cysteine and asparagine concentrations (lower panel), whereas the concentrations of leucine and most other amino acids showed only moderate (and statistically insignificant) changes (upper panel) (107).

concentration. High-pressure liquid chromatography has confirmed the age-related decrease in mean plasma cysteine concentration (173).

As cysteine and asparagine are protein-forming amino acids, the body always has a large reservoir of both amino acids. In healthy, young individuals, adequate amounts of free amino acids are maintained even under starving (postabsorptive) conditions through the mechanism of autophagy, as discussed previously. The concomitant decrease in both cysteine and asparagine in old age is therefore best interpreted as another manifestation of the age-related decline in autophagic protein catabolism (chapter one). Cysteine and asparagine are affected more strongly than most other amino acids because they are represented in the plasma at a much lower concentration (twelve micromolar (μM) and sixty μM, respectively), whereas their representation in muscle proteins is in the same order of magnitude as that of other amino acids. The absence or presence of autophagic muscle protein breakdown is therefore expected to affect the plasma cysteine and asparagine concentrations to a greater relative extent (percentage) than most other amino acids.

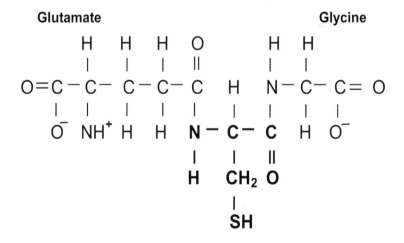

Fig. 7. Chemical structure of glutathione. Glutathione is a tripeptide consisting of glutamate, cysteine, and glycine. Its function as an antioxidant and radical scavenger is essentially based on the sulfhydryl group (SH) of the cysteine moiety.

The amino acid cysteine is the most limiting precursor for the biosynthesis of glutathione. This tripeptide (figure 7) is the quantitatively most important scavenger of free radicals and an important substrate for the removal of hydrogen peroxide. In line with the circadian diet-dependent variation in plasma cysteine concentrations, the glutathione concentration in the liver and plasma show a strong circadian variation and an even stronger decrease by 50 percent or more upon extensive starvation (35, 169). It has therefore been suggested that cells and tissues may be most vulnerable in the postabsorptive state; and the greatest impact of oxidative stress on aging-related parameters in man is likely to take place at night and in the early morning hours (107).

In line with the age-related decrease in plasma cysteine concentrations in man (figure 6), an age-related decrease in the intracellular glutathione concentration has been reported for the liver and kidney from rats (11), brain tissues from rats and mice (68, 280, 308), retinal glia cells from guinea pigs (274), and spleen cells from mice (133). In mice, intravenous injection of cysteine derivatives, such as N-acetylcysteine or glutathione, was shown to cause a significant increase in the hepatic glutathione concentration within two hours (169), indicating the hepatic glutathione concentration is largely determined by the availability of its precursor amino acid cysteine.

Data on the age-related changes in glutathione levels in different tissues in humans are presently not available. In view of the entire wealth of available information, it may be reasonable to assume:

1. The age-related decrease in autophagic activity leads to a shift in amino acid homeostasis, as manifested in the decrease in postabsorptive plasma cysteine and asparagine levels.

2. The decrease in postabsorptive cysteine eventually causes a decrease in intracellular glutathione levels and corresponding increase in oxidative stress (reviewed in 107).

3. The age-related decrease in glutathione concentrations and corresponding increase in ROS levels inevitably render elderly subjects increasingly vulnerable to oxidation and changes in redox-sensitive signaling pathways (102, 103, 106)

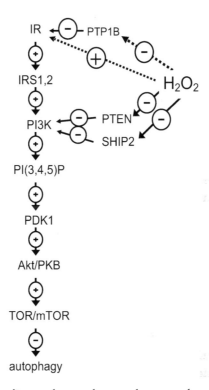

Fig. 8. Insulin signaling pathways that regulate autophagy. Binding of insulin leads to autophosphorylation and activation of the insulin receptor (IR) kinase and recruitment of insulin-receptor substrates (IRS-1, IRS-2). Phosphatidyl-ionsitol 3-kinase (PI3K) converts phosphatidylinositol (4,5) diphosphate (PI(4,5)P2) into phosphatidylinositol (3,4,5) triphosphate (PI(3,4,5)P3. This binds and activates phosphoinositide-dependent protein kinase 1 (PDK1), which phosphorylates the serine/threonine kinase Akt1. Akt1 is activated by binding to PI(3,4,5) P3 at the cell membrane and subsequent phosphorylation. Akt1 stimulates the target of rapamycin (TOR or the mammalian mTOR), an inhibitor of autophagy. Insulin receptor signaling activity is downregulated by protein tyrosine phosphatase 1B (PTB1B), which dephosphorylates the IR kinase domain, and the phosphatase and tensine homologue on chromosome 10 (PTEN) and SH2 domain-containing inositol phosphatase (SHIP2), both of which dephosphorylate PI(3,4,5)P3. Hydrogen peroxide enhances the autophosphorylation of IR kinase and inhibits the activity of the three phosphatases.

and facilitate the development of secondary oxidative stress by various disease-related mechanisms of ROS production, as discussed later.

Effect of oxidative stress on the insulin receptor signaling cascade

As the autophagic activity is negatively regulated by the insulin receptor signaling cascade and amino acid concentrations (figure 3), autophagy is maximally derepressed under starving conditions when amino acid concentrations and insulin levels are low. But, even in the absence of insulin, the basic activity of the insulin receptor signaling pathway is abnormally increased by oxidative stress. The age-related increase in oxidative stress and its effect on the insulin receptor signaling pathway provide a simple explanation for the age-related change in the homeostatic control of cysteine and asparagine.

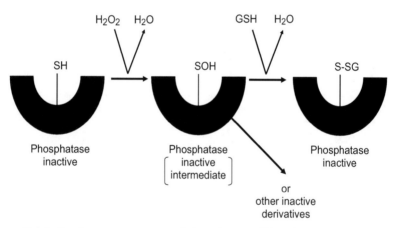

Fig. 9. Oxidative inactivation of phosphatases. Phosphatases typically contain an SH group at their catalytic center. Upon oxidation by hydrogen peroxide, the phosphatase is converted into a catalytically inactive intermediate and other inactive derivatives, such as the mixed glutathione disulfide (S-SG).

Activation of the insulin receptor involves its autophosphorylation, and it is typically followed by phosphorylation of several target proteins in the signaling cascade (figure 8). Activation of this cascade is negatively regulated by several phosphatases, including protein tyrosine phosphatase 1B (PTB 1B), phosphatase and tensin homologue on chromosome 10 (PTEN), and SH2-domain-containing inositol phosphatase (SHIP2), all of which are inactivated even under moderately oxidative conditions (24, 25, 34, 27, 119, 137, 306). Phosphatases typically contain a sulfhydryl group in their catalytic domain, which is converted by hydrogen peroxide into a sulfenic acid moiety. This oxidation renders these enzymes catalytically inactive (figure 9). In contrast to the functional inactivation of the phosphatases, the basic insulin receptor tyrosine kinase activity itself is strongly increased by low concentrations of hydrogen peroxide or an oxidative shift in the glutathione redox status (312). As this effect of hydrogen peroxide acts directly on the cytoplasmic domain, it activates the insulin receptor kinase domain, even in the absence of insulin. Ultimately, the activity of the insulin receptor signaling pathway is determined by the balance between kinase and phosphatase activities. The oxidative activation of the kinase—together with the inactivation of the phosphatases—tends to enhance synergistically the activity of this signaling pathway.

Several recent studies illustrate the in vivo relevance of these regulatory processes. Treatment of mice with cysteine or N-acetylcysteine for a period of one week was shown to cause a strong dose-dependent increase in plasma glucose concentration (360). In another study in mice, overexpression of the hydrogen peroxide scavenging enzyme glutathione peroxidase 1 (GPX1) was shown to decrease the autophosphorylation of the hepatic insulin receptor and clearance of glucose from the blood (241). In line with these findings, a recent study in pregnant women revealed a significant correlation between increased glutathione peroxidase activity and decreased glucose clearance (69). Between the time of entry and third trimester of pregnancy, the women showed an increase in glutathione peroxidase activity and concomitant increase in postabsorptive insulin and glucose concentrations. Individual changes in insulin and glucose levels were significantly correlated with the individual changes in glutathione peroxidase. A similar increase in postabsorptive insulin and glucose levels, indicating a decreased basic insulin receptor signaling activity, was observed in young, obese, nondiabetic women after oral supplementation of N-acetylcysteine (159).

Together with the mechanisms described previously, the redox sensitivity of the insulin receptor signaling cascade constitutes a vicious cycle of progressive oxidative stress in aging (figure 5) (reviewed in 107).

Chapter Three

Further Evidence for the Role of the Vicious Cycle

Life Span Extension in Animals with Increased Scavenging Activity for Hydrogen Peroxide and Oxygen Radicals

The schematic illustration in figure 5 explains in a slightly simplified form the seemingly paradoxical finding that animal mutants with an impairment of the insulin signaling mechanism live substantially longer than their normal counterparts. But figure 5 also shows that oxygen radicals and/or hydrogen peroxide and their effect on the activation of the insulin signaling mechanism play a key role in this cycle. It is therefore not unexpected to see the life span is similarly increased by mutations that decrease the levels of oxygen radicals and hydrogen peroxide. Specifically, an increased expression of the enzymes superoxide dismutase (SOD) and catalase, which degrade oxygen radicals and hydrogen peroxide, respectively, were shown to be involved in the life span extension of several strains of worms and flies. These enzymes occur normally in practically all tissues of man and animals, but they are obviously not always present in sufficient amounts.

A group of proteins called FOXO play a particularly important role in this context. Members of this group of proteins exist in many species, including man. Life span extension in worms with a mutation in the insulin signaling mechanism was found to require not only an intact autophagic mechanism but also the FOXO protein of the worms. Like autophagy, FOXO protein activity is downregulated by the insulin signaling mechanism (figure 10). As FOXO proteins stimulate the expression of the oxygen radical scavenger, SOD, and the hydrogen peroxide-degrading enzyme, catalase, FOXO proteins may be considered as an integral part of the vicious cycle (figure 10). In flies, overexpression of the FOXO protein was shown to be sufficient for life span extension and prevented the age-related decline in cardiac function. In addition, mammalian FOXO proteins upregulate different mechanisms of protein degradation, including autophagy. This effect is likely to contribute to the plasma cysteine homeostasis (figure 10). A more detailed explanation of the complex interactions in figure 10 will be discussed later.

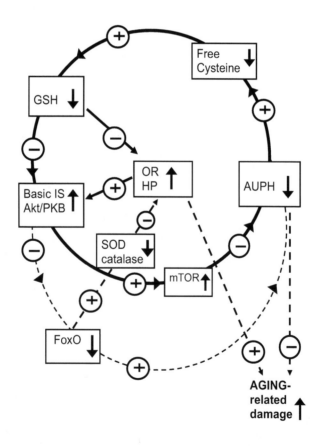

Fig.10. Effect of FOXO proteins on the vicious cycle of oxidative stress. The FOXO proteins are transcription factors, which (like autophagy) are negatively regulated by the insulin signaling cascade through the Akt kinase and optimally activated during periods of starvation. An abnormal increase in basal insulin signaling and Akt activity negatively affects the activity of the FOXO proteins. In worms, the FOXO homologue DAF-16 was shown to positively regulate the expression of superoxide dismutase and catalase, that is, enzymes involved in the removal of oxygen radicals and hydrogen peroxide, respectively (reviewed in 303). The mammalian homologues FOXO-1 and FOXO-3 were shown to induce the expression of proteins involved in both autophagic and non-autophagic mechanisms of protein breakdown. The non-autophagic mechanism contributes to the degradation of damaged, long-lived skeletal muscle proteins that are not degraded by the autophagic mechanism. In fruit flies, overexpression of FOXO was shown to prevent the age-related decline in cardiac function and increased the life span. Various other aging-related functions of FOXO proteins are presently being studied.

Oxidative Stress as a Major Cause of Aging-related Structural Damage

There is an increasing public awareness of *oxygen radicals* and *oxidative stress* as putative mediators of aging. Oxygen radicals are the most prominent subgroup among the more widely known free radicals. The idea that radical-mediated oxidative stress may play a key role in the mechanism of aging has indeed been proposed more than fifty years ago, and a wealth of evidence now suggests that oxidative damage in all major constituents of cells and tissues increases with age. Among other tissues, an increase in protein oxidation has been demonstrated in various brain regions and notably in the hippocampus, the major site of memory function. Quite possibly, the age-related increase in oxidative tissue damage may be as important as the age-related decline in autophagic activity as a life span determining factor. Interestingly, studies on the effects of the antioxidative vitamins A, C, or E on aging-related degenerative processes essentially revealed no significant effects. Supplementation of these antioxidants during the day may have indeed very little effect on the decline of the intracellular glutathione concentration during the postabsorptive period in the night and on the resulting aberrant activation of the insulin signaling mechanism. In contrast, supplementation of the glutathione precursor cysteine has yielded a number of promising results that will be discussed later.

Life Span Extension by Calorie Restriction

Calorie restriction (partial starvation) is known to extend the life span of almost all species tested so far, including invertebrates, fish, and mammals. Weindruch and Walford have used the term *undernutrition without malnutrition* to emphasize the need that all essential nutrients should be provided in adequate amounts. The mechanism by which calorie restriction causes life span extension has been the subject of numerous investigations, but it is still not completely understood. Studies in animals have shown that calorie restriction has an impact on all major elements of the vicious cycle (figure 5). Specifically, life span extension in diet-restricted animals was found to be associated with increased blood glutathione levels, increased autophagic activity, and decreased oxidative tissue damage. Calorie restriction is a promising intervention in attempts to extend the life span of man and has been included in the guidelines described in addendum one.

Impact of the Vicious Cycle on the Frequency of Major Aging-related Diseases

As the average human life span is largely determined by aging-related diseases, such as cardiovascular diseases, at least some of these diseases are directly affected by the mechanisms discussed previously. Abnormally large amounts of oxygen radicals are produced in various human diseases, including cardiovascular diseases by disease-specific mechanisms. At face value, these mechanisms of oxidative stress appear to be unrelated to the vicious cycle in figure 5. However, as the age-related decrease in glutathione concentration compromises the capacity to scavenge oxygen radicals and hydrogen peroxide, this decrease also aggravates the disease-related mechanisms of oxidative stress and explains the incidence of oxidative stress-related diseases increases with age.

Studies on skeletal muscle wasting in primates and mice have indicated that an insufficient availability of cysteine in the liver is associated with an increased breakdown of amino acids and their conversion into urea. In mice, cysteine supplementation reversed this process. This mechanism potentially aggravates the negative consequences of the cycle in figure 5/figure 10.

Inflammation as a Consequence of Oxidative Stress

Aging is associated with increased levels of certain inflammatory cytokines (which are hormone-like proteins) such as tumor necrosis factor α (TNFα) and Interleukin 6 (IL-6). It may therefore be viewed as a low-grade inflammatory condition. The two transcription factors, NF-κB and AP-1 which induce the production of various inflammatory cytokines are activated by oxidative stress. It is therefore reasonable to assume that the age-related increase in inflammatory cytokines is facilitated by the age-related decrease in glutathione levels and the resulting oxidative stress. In elderly persons, high plasma TNFα levels are correlated with increased morbidity and mortality.

Seemingly Paradoxical Role of Oxidative Stress in Insulin Resistance and Type 2 Diabetes

At face value it was a surprising finding that the impairment of the insulin signaling cascade caused an increase in life span in mice, flies and worms whereas in clinical medicine even a partial loss of insulin responsiveness is known to cause type 2 diabetes, a potentially deadly disease (see chapter one). Another surprising finding was that insulin responsiveness is inhibited under reducing conditions through the increased activity of several phosphatases (chapter two), and paradoxically also inhibited under conditions of oxidative stress through the oxidative induction of NF-κB and TNFα which cause the inhibition of insulin receptor substrate 1 (IRS-1). Antioxidants have in fact been used in the treatment of diabetic patients to enhance insulin responsiveness. In the end, oxidative stress causes a low ratio of signal to background noise in the insulin signaling cascade because the physiological response to insulin is impaired at the level of IRS-1 whereas the insulin independent background activity is abnormally increased by the inhibition of the phosphatases that act downstream of IRS-1. Because studies have shown that the transport of creatine from the blood into the tissues is stimulated by insulin, diabetic persons are also expected to have relatively low phosphocreatine levels which may additionally impair insulin signaling. Refilling the tissue creatine pool may be a major challenge.

Scientific Evidence

Genetic studies linking life span to the expression of enzymes that remove superoxide radicals and/or hydrogen peroxide

Several longevity strains of roundworms and fruit flies collectively suggest that an increase in oxidative stress resistance is often associated with an increase in life span. Specifically, an increase in the superoxide radical removing enzyme superoxide dismutase (Mn-SOD) has been implicated in life span extension in the daf-2 mutant of *C. elegans* (162). The hydrogen peroxide-degrading enzyme catalase was shown to be required for life span extension in daf-C and clk-1 mutants in *C. elegans* (345). In the common fruit fly, an increased life span was found in strains with extra copies of genes of SOD and catalase (269, 282). The long-living mth mutant of the common fruit fly was shown to have an increased resistance to a free radical generator (221). Also, in the p66shc mouse mutant, an increased life span was associated with an increased resistance to oxidative stress (248). A significantly increased life span was also found in genetically manipulated mice with increased, but otherwise normally regulated levels of Arf and p53 proteins (237). This strain of mice contains significantly increased glutathione levels in the liver, decreased ROS levels in the spleen, and decreased levels of lipid peroxidation in the liver.

Comparative studies on eight mammalian species have also shown a strong correlation between the maximum life span of these species and capacity of their cells (skin fibroblasts and lymphocytes) to withstand hydrogen peroxide and other forms of oxidative stress (177).

A special case in point is the role of transcription factors of the FOXO family in longevity mutants. In worms, DAF-16 stimulates, among other aging-related genes, the expression of the genes of SOD and catalase, that is, proteins involved in the removal of superoxide and hydrogen peroxide, respectively (303) (figure 10). The mammalian FOXO-3a was shown to stimulate the expression of MnSOD (196, 217). As FOXO transcription factors are also downregulated by the insulin receptor signaling pathway and derepressed under conditions of starvation, the FOXO proteins may be considered as integral components of the vicious cycle, that is, first cause of death, as illustrated in figure 10.

Oxidative stress as a cause of aging-related structural and functional damage

The hypothesis that oxygen radical-mediated tissue damage may play a major role in aging has been proposed more than fifty years ago (148). Work by many laboratories and in different species has shown that lipid peroxidation and oxidative damage of proteins and DNA increase with age (19, 56, 57, 73, 121, 140, 145,166, 179, 215, 225, 258, 266, 288, 297, 330, 333, 356, 361, 388). This increase in oxidative damage is generally associated with a corresponding decrease in the concentrations of antioxidants, such as serumand tissue levels of vitamin E, plasma concentrations of vitamin C (19, 92, 200, 315), and intracellular glutathione concentrations in various tissues from rats, mice, and guinea pigs (11, 133, 273, 274, 280, 308).

The age-related increase in oxidative brain damage is again best exemplified by products of lipid peroxidation (140, 73, 258, 266, 57, 297, 388), protein oxidation (333, 328, 288), and DNA modification (145). An increase in protein oxidation has been demonstrated in various brain regions, including the hippocampus as the major site of memory function (328). A decrease in glutathione concentration or glutathione redox status was also found in all mammalian brain regions tested, including the hippocampus (57, 97, 388).

But levels of oxidative damage do not always strictly correlate with differences in life span. The naked mole rat, for example, is exceptionally long-lived in comparison to mammals of similar size, but, surprisingly, it has exceptionally high levels of oxidative damage (9). Even more strikingly, mice heterozygous for the SOD2 gene were shown to have reduced MnSOD activity (50 percent) in all tissues throughout life and significantly increased levels of DNA damage in all tissues tested, but normal mean and maximum life spans (362). These findings may be best explained by the fact that the two most prominent ROS, superoxide and hydrogen peroxide, have very different properties and biological effects. The more long-lived hydrogen peroxide travels greater distances, and it is typically detoxified by catalase and glutathione peroxidase, which requires glutathione as a cosubstrate. A reduction in the essentially mitochondrial MnSOD is expected to increase steady state levels of superoxide but decrease steady state levels of the long-lived and far-traveling hydrogen peroxide. A partial reduction in MnSOD levels may not necessarily enhance the progression of the cycle in figure 5. There is a strong possibility that the ROS-mediated dysregulation of redox-sensitive signaling pathways may have an even more important effect on aging than the ROS-mediated oxidative damage of cellular constituents (101). Changes in MnSOD levels and the resulting changes in steady state levels of hydrogen peroxide may have a particularly strong impact on the set points of redox-sensitive signaling pathways, including the insulin receptor signaling mechanism in figure 5.

Life span extension by calorie restriction

Calorie restriction is a method of partial starvation that has been shown to increase the life span in various animal species (332, 373). In some studies, calorie restriction was shown to increase autophagic activity (99, 254, 64). In several studies of mice, rats, and fruit flies, life span extension of calorie-restricted animals was associated with a decrease in oxidative tissue damage (145, 387). This series of independent studies of different parameters of the vicious cycle of figure 5 indicates that calorie restriction improves the general status of this cycle. Although the effects of caloric restriction on the quality of life and the life span of man have not been systematically studied, some humans voluntarily practice calorie restriction. Weindruch and Walford (372) have described a detailed guideline for the use of calorie restriction in man.

Facilitation of oxidative stress in aging-related diseases in humans

The age-related decrease in glutathione concentration inevitably compromises the ROS scavenging capacity and facilitates certain secondary disease-related mechanism of oxidative stress. An important case in point is the group of cardiovascular diseases that account for a high percentage of human mortality. A critical step in the pathogenesis of atherosclerosis is the impairment of endothelial function (6, 281), which is typically associated with increased oxidative stress (138, 300, 302, 355). Disease-related mechanisms of oxidative stress, such as xanthine oxidase-dependent ROS production or aberrant NADPH oxidase-mediated ROS production, are inevitably aggravated by the age-related decrease in glutathione levels, thus explaining the age-related increase in the incidence of cardiovascular diseases. On average, patients with cardiovascular disease show an oxidative shift in the plasma thiol-disulfide redox status (120, 174). Atrial fibrillation was shown to be associated with an oxidative shift in both plasma cysteine and glutathione redox status (263). Finally, in middle-aged individuals at risk of cardiovascular disease, a change in carotid intima media thickness was found to be directly correlated with an oxidative shift in glutathione redox status (15, 175). Other examples have been reviewed elsewhere (107).

Aging and inflammation

The aging process may be viewed as a low-grade inflammatory condition (45). The age-related increase in the steady state level of IL-6 mRNA and IL-6 production in the brain (297) is a well documented example. In vivo and in vitro studies have indicated that the increase in IL-6 expression results at least to some extent from the enhanced binding of NF-κB to the IL-6 promotor, and NF-κB has also been implicated in the upregulation of TNFα and IL-8 in human dendritic cells under oxidative conditions (reviewed in 106). The two transcription factors NF-κB and AP-1 are activated by ROS and also by an oxidative shift in the glutathione redox status (reviewed in 102). It is therefore reasonable to assume that the age-related increase in inflammatory cytokines is facilitated by the age-related decrease in glutathione levels. Both NF-κB and TNFα have also been implicated in the development of inflammation-associated cancer (reviewed in 106,107).

Effect of cysteine availability on urea cycle activity in catabolic conditions

Several studies in different species suggested an insufficient availability of cysteine may also lead to an increase in hepatic urea production and negative nitrogen balance, implying a loss of amino acids. The catabolism of amino acids is determined, at least to some extent, by the rate at which ammonium ions in the liver are converted into either urea or glutamine. Whereas glutamine biosynthesis is essentially neutral, urea production requires hydrogen carbonate ions (HCO_3^-) and indirectly generates protons (reviewed in 105). The production of carbamoylphosphate as the rate-limiting step in urea biosynthesis is limited by the availability of HCO_3^- ions, which are scavenged by protons. In line with this mechanism, several independent studies have indicated that the hepatic cysteine catabolism into sulfate and protons controls urea production in favor of glutamine biosynthesis, thereby retaining the nitrogen in the amino acid reservoir (141, 190, 139, 108). Increased hepatic urea concentrations and urea/glutamine ratios were found to be correlated with decreased hepatic sulfate levels and plasma cyst(e)ine levels in SIV-infected rhesus macaques and tumor-bearing mice (139, 109, 141). In mice, cysteine supplementation reversed these changes (141). Cytokines may play an important role in the dysregulation of urea production as a similar increase in hepatic urea/glutamine ratios and decrease in hepatic sulfate levels was induced in mice after treatment with Interleukin-6 (141). Taken together, these findings suggest the decreased availability of cysteine may have a negative effect on the nitrogen balance and this effect is independent of (and additive to) the oxidative stress-related effects discussed previously.

Chapter Four

The Emerging Paradigm

Taken together, scientific studies from different fields of research strongly suggest that life span is critically influenced by a mechanism of controlled self-destruction called autophagy. Autophagy is an ancient biological mechanism for the removal of cellular waste and maintenance of adequate free amino acid levels under starving conditions (amino acid homeostasis). Research in various laboratories has shown that autophagic activity decreases with age, cellular waste accumulates in old age, and amino acid homeostasis also changes with age. The aberrant stimulation of the insulin signaling mechanism in the starved state by oxygen radicals and hydrogen peroxide, the downregulation of autophagic activity by this signaling mechanism, and the resulting decrease in the postabsorptive (starved) plasma cysteine and intracellular glutathione levels constitute a vicious cycle of progressive oxidative stress (figure 5/figure 10). This mechanism provides a simple and plausible explanation for the age-related decline in autophagic activity. As the accumulation of cellular waste, a decrease in cellular glutathione concentrations, and various manifestations of age-related oxidative stress are common hallmarks of aging in a broad range of species tested so far, the oxidative spiral in figure 5/figure 10 may be viewed as the cycle of the first cause of death. Based on these findings, there is reason to believe that both the life span and quality of life in old age can be increased by practical interventions designed to reestablish adequate levels of autophagic waste recycling and postabsorptive cysteine concentrations. It would be unwise to ignore this opportunity.

Chapter Five

Primary Interventions

Life Span Extending Drugs: Rapamycin as a Case in Point

The possibility that life span extending drugs for humans are within reach is strongly supported by the recent report by Harrison,D.E., R. Strong, Z.D. Scharp, J.F. Nelson, C.M. Astle, K. Flurkey, N.L. Nadon, J.E. Wilkinson, K. Frenkel, C.S. Carter, M. Pahor, M.A. Javors, E. Fernandez, and R.A. Miller. 2009. Rapamycin fed late in life extends lifespan in genetically heterogeneous mice. *Nature* 460:392-395. Because interventions that delay aging would greatly benefit health and quality of life in old age, the U.S. National Institute's on Aging Interventions Testing Program ITP) has been established to test compounds of interest for their effects on life span in mice. The first and only compound that was found to robustly increase life span in three independent research centers was rapamycin. It was quite satisfying to see that this life span extending effect was demonstrable even in mice which started receiving this drug at 600 days of age corresponding to 60 years in humans. As this compound is known to inhibit the target of rapamycin (TOR/mTOR in mammals), which is a key element in the insulin signaling cascade (see figure 3), rapamycin was indeed expected to inhibit the oxidative spiral in figure 5/figure 10 and to have similar effects as the mutations described in chapter one. Its life span extending effect provides additional support for the concepts and conclusions outlined in the previous chapters.

However, the insulin signaling cascade and its key element, mTOR, are not only devils that shorten life span but have important positive functions in the metabolic (mostly synthetic) response to food intake (see figure 3). As discussed in chapter one and chapter two, silencing of mTOR is most critically needed in the starved condition (that is in humans during the night) and not after food intake. To avoid potential adverse effects of rapamycin after food intake (that is in the postprandial period) one may consider supplementation of low doses of rapamycin in humans at night before sleeping. In any case, one would like to see at first clinical studies on safety.

Calorie Restriction

As already discussed in chapter 3, dietary restriction was shown to increase the life span in several animal species and improve the status of the vicious cycle of figure 5, as judged by the increase in autophagic activity, the increase in glutathione concentration, and less pronounced manifestations of oxidative stress. Although a positive effect of calorie restriction on the quality of life in old age or life span of man has not been demonstrated, calorie restriction is also voluntarily practiced among humans. It would be unwise to ignore the potential benefits of this method. Recommendations for the practical application of calorie restrictions in humans have been described by Weindruch and Walford (372) in considerable detail. These authors especially emphasized the need for adequate amounts of essential nutrients, notably zinc, vitamin E, copper, magnesium, iron, niacin, vitamin B12, pantothenic acid, calcium, riboflavin, folacin, vitamin A, vitamin B6, thiamine, and vitamin C. They also suggested that calorie restriction should not be used during childhood and the reduction in calorie intake should be individualized to account for the interindividual variation in energy metabolism. For the United States population, a daily calorie intake of around eighteen hundred to two thousand kilocalories has been recommended as most appropriate (see 372). It has also been recommended to adjust the protein intake to approximately 0.8 to 1.0 gram per kilogram of body weight per day to avoid malnutrition while aiming for undernutrition (372).

For someone who is prepared to follow such a rigorous protocol of calorie restriction, it is recommended to look into the specialized literature on dietary restriction (see 372 and Walford,R.L., D. Mock, R. Verdery, and T. MacCallum. 2002. Calorie restriction in Biosphere 2: Alterations in physiologic, hematologic, hormonal, and biochemical parameters in humans restricted for a 2-years period. *J Gerontol* 57A:B211-B224). However, such a rigorous form of calorie restriction may not find many afficionados and may not even be necessary. As aging is typically associated with an undesirable loss of skeletal muscle mass and muscle function, calorie restriction may only be used to the point where the skeletal muscle is not negatively affected. There are reasons to believe that a less rigorous program of calorie restriction in man may still have a positive effect on the vicious cycle of figure 5, as concluded from a study on nondiabetic, obese persons. It is recommended that alternating periods of moderate calorie restriction may be combined with other interventions as described in addendum one.

Antioxidant vitamins

To deal with the effects of oxygen radicals and oxidative stress on aging most books generally refer to the use of antioxidant vitamins. Treatment of age-related or disease-related oxidative stress with supplements of antioxidant vitamins may seem to be a trivial affair, but several clinical studies on the effects of antioxidant vitamins yielded less than impressive effects. Most people normally consume sufficient amounts of vitamins with their diet or as vitamin supplements. A further increase in vitamin intake is unlikely to increase the maximum human lifespan. One may want to keep in mind that oxygen radicals in adequate and well regulated amounts are needed as mediators in signaling processes.

Cysteine Supplementation to Decrease the Oxidative Stress

Cysteine supplementation is a special case of antioxidant intervention because cysteine is the most limiting biosynthetic precursor of glutathione which is the quantitatively most important intracellular antioxidant and radical scavenger in the body. At face value, it appears that the most obvious way to compensate for the aging-related decrease

41

in plasma cysteine and intracellular glutathione concentrations is to increase the dietary intake of cysteine-rich foods or supplements. As low glutathione levels and a corresponding increase in oxidative stress favor the aberrant activation of the insulin signaling mechanism and decrease in autophagic activity (chapter 2), dietary cysteine supplementation is expected to break the oxidative spiral of figure 5/figure 10, at least to some extent. In using cysteine as an antioxidant supplement one should take into account, however, that the metabolic utilization of cysteine is remarkably complex (see scientific evidence). Practical guidelines are described in addendum one.

Until now, the effect of cysteine supplementation on the autophagic activity has not been demonstrated because it is difficult to measure autophagy without invasive techniques. A few clinical studies have shown that cysteine supplementation does have the desired effect on this oxidative spiral. In one study, supplementation of the cysteine derivative N-acetylcysteine has caused a significant decrease in the basic insulin responsiveness in the postabsorptive state, as indicated by the fasted plasma glucose and insulin concentrations. In another study on frail, elderly patients, N-acetylcysteine supplementation was shown to increase muscle strength during a six-week period of physical exercise. In the absence of cysteine supplementation, the benefits from the exercise program in terms of muscle strength were significantly correlated with the quality of amino acid homeostasis, as indicated by the plasma concentrations of cysteine and asparagine. On the average, the exercise program was completely ineffective in persons who had low plasma concentrations of cysteine and asparagine under starving conditions. Conversely, persons with low cysteine and asparagine levels showed the greatest benefits from cysteine supplementation. Two other clinical studies have shown that supplementation with high doses of a cysteine-rich whey protein in combination with resistance exercise yielded a significantly greater improvement in muscle strength than supplementation with a placebo or a protein low in cysteine. Because the cysteine-rich whey protein contains many amino acids other than cysteine, supplementation with N-acetylcysteine has the advantage that it directly demonstrates the effects of cysteine. However, the use of a cysteine-rich protein such as whey protein may be the better alternative for long-term cysteine supplementation over many months or years (chapter 8).

In view of the vicious cycle of the decreasing autophagic activity, decreasing postabsorptive cysteine and glutathione levels, and corresponding increase in aberrant insulin signaling activity (figure 5), there was the theoretical possibility that a sufficient increase in dietary cysteine intake may increase the autophagic activity to the extent it will generate enough cysteine from endogeneous protein sources to maintain amino acid homeostasis and the postabsorptive concentration of plasma cysteine at a youthful level. However, the amount of cysteine supplementation that had been given to the frail, elderly patients was sufficient to detectably increase muscle strength but not the postabsorptive plasma cysteine and asparagine concentrations in the early morning.

In contrast to the scarcity of clinical trials on cysteine supplementation in man, there are many reports on the effects of N-acetylcysteine on the aging-related functional decline in animals. As the cognitive decline is one of the most devastating consequences of aging, it was particularly interesting to see that cysteine supplementation reduces the rate of oxidative damage in the brain and ameliorates the decline of memory functions and various biochemical functions.

Excessive cysteine intake may have several potentially adverse effects. One of the major adverse effects is the formation of excessive metabolic acid (chapter 7). Cysteine supplementation should therefore be used in a balanced way. The intracellular concentrations of the cysteine derivative, glutathione, can only be increased up to a certain point. Any excess of cysteine is broken down into products, some of which are metabolic acids. The effect of acid formation on the hepatic urea cycle and its consequences for the plasma amino acid levels have been described in detail in the science section of chapter 3. In principle, acid formation can be neutralized by an adequate consumption of fruit, vegetables, or citric acid salts, as described subsequently. But an unnecessarily high cysteine intake should clearly be avoided. Because the main cysteine-rich protein sources, such as meat, eggs, and milk products, typically contain a substantial amount of fat, the most trivial adverse effect of these cysteine sources is the high fat intake. This problem can be avoided by focusing on cysteine sources that contain less fat.

Water-assisted autophagy: A novel Intervention Acting on the Target of Rapamycin

The concentration of the regulatory amino acids, which downregulate the autophagic activity (figure 3), is one of the most attractive targets in attempts to enhance this activity. The term *water-assisted autophagy* describes a mild and simple method designed to increase the autophagic activity by drinking one hundred to five hundred milliliters in the night about two to three hours before breakfast in order to temporarily dilute the regulatory amino acids in the blood plasma. *Water-assisted autophagy* is designed to act upon mTOR, that is the same regulatory element which is targeted by rapamycin. The temporary derepression of autophagy is expected to cause the release of free amino acids, notably from the muscle tissue, up to the point where the original equilibrium of the regulatory amino acids in the blood is reestablished. The temporary stimulation of autophagy is expected to cause a relatively high proportional increase in the plasma cysteine concentration, as described subsequently.

As autophagy is a method of controlled self-destruction, it is not surprising that the use of larger amounts of water (five hundred milliliters) was occasionally found to be associated with a sensation of stress. This feeling of stress may serve as a guideline to determine the acceptable amount of water. Generally, drinking this amount of clean water is considered as safe.

The strong point of this method is its simplicity. The scientific principle of this method is based on solid science. But its effect still needs to be systematically investigated, and the most suitable amount of water remains to be determined. Also, this method may be subject to interference by an aberrant activation of the insulin receptor signaling mechanism, which is likely to occur under the increasingly oxidative conditions of the aging organism. This method should therefore be combined with a program of cysteine supplementation.

Scientific Evidence

Calorie restriction as a strategy known to extend life span in animals

The effect of caloric restriction on the median or maximum life span has been extensively investigated in numerous species for many decades (reviewed in 372, 373, 364). It is the only well-established interventional strategy known to extend the life span in a broad range of animals. However, dietary restriction was found to have a lesser effect on longevity in wild mice than in laboratory strains, and the interim results from two ongoing

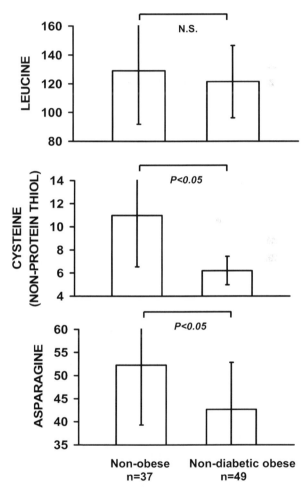

Fig. 11. Fasting plasma amino acid concentrations (μM±S.D.) in nonobese and obese women. The data shows the postabsorptive plasma asparagine, cysteine, and leucine concentrations of thirty- to sixty-nine-year-old nonobese or obese, nondiabetic women (W. Dröge, unpublished observation).

studies in rhesus monkeys are still preliminary (reviewed in 364) but start to yield very promising results (R.J. Colman et al. 2009. Caloric restriction delays disease onset and mortality in rhesus monkeys. *Science* 325:201-204.) It is also fair to state that rigorous calorie restriction in humans is associated with a substantial amount of sacrifice. Consequently, a program of rigorous calorie restriction may seem appealing to some, but certainly not to the majority of our society. Also, rigorous calorie restriction is likely to cause frequent periods of low plasma glucose levels, that is, so-called episodes of hypoglycemia, which are known to induce hypoglycemic response factors such as cortisol, glucagon, and adrenaline (epinephrine). The combination of these hypoglycemic hormones has strong catabolic effects on skeletal muscle protein involving the proteasomal mechanism of proteolysis (76). Because plasma glucocorticoid levels increase in many catabolic conditions, it has been suggested that glucocorticoids may generally play an important role in skeletal muscle wasting (76, 115, 151, 216). This raises the question whether calorie restriction may still be effective in terms of life span extension and improved quality of life in old age if practiced at a more moderate level just below the point where one would start to compromise body cell mass, muscle mass, and muscle function. Unfortunately, no systematic studies are available that would answer this question, but there is preliminary information to suggest that it does. A study of the postabsorptive plasma cysteine, asparagine, and leucine concentrations (that is, key parameters to determine the status of amino acid homeostasis and the vicious cycle of figure 5) has shown that nondiabetic, obese women had significantly decreased plasma cysteine and asparagine levels compared to nonobese control women of similar age (figure 11). In general, these obese women had gained in body weight by excessive consumption of carbohydrates. If one considers this eating habit as a form of negative calorie restriction, one is led to believe that calorie restriction at all levels within a relatively wide range may still provide benefits with regard to the cycle in figure 5. Of course, this point needs further investigation. If this point is confirmed, everybody may find his or her personal level of calorie restriction.

Cysteine supplementation to target the aberrant insulin receptor signaling activity and ameliorate the oxidative stress

As a decrease in intracellular glutathione or increase in oxidative stress causes an aberrant activation of the insulin receptor signaling pathway in the absence of insulin, and the insulin receptor signaling cascade suppresses the autophagic activity, cysteine supplementation was expected to break the oxidative spiral of figure 5/figure 10. One clinical study in obese, non-diabetic women has already shown that supplementation of N-acetylcysteine at the relatively low dose of 1.8 grams per day corresponding to a daily dose of 1.4 grams cysteine caused the desired significant decrease in the basal insulin responsiveness in the fasted state (159).

A few clinical studies have shown that cysteine supplementation exerts positive effects on several functional parameters, which typically deteriorate in old age and may be viewed as surrogate parameters of aging. The most debilitating aging-related changes are the cognitive decline and massive loss of muscle mass and muscle function. In contrast to the former, the latter provides relatively robust endpoints that can be measured with good precision and reproducibility in kilograms, centimeters, and seconds. The loss of muscle function in old age has also received much attention because it is associated with psychological stress, loss of social functions, financial burden, and increased probability of death (292). A placebo-controlled study in frail, elderly patients has shown that N-acetylcysteine treatment at a daily dose of 1.8 grams doubled the increase in knee extension strength during a six-week program of physical exercise (152). In addition, it slowed the subsequent decline in muscle strength during the six-week follow-up period after discontinuation of the exercise program. The explorative analysis of this study revealed the mean of the exercise-induced changes in the placebo group was significantly correlated with the postabsorptive plasma concentrations of cysteine and asparagine, indicating a direct relationship between exercise benefits and plasma amino acid homeostasis. Importantly, this association between exercise benefit and plasma amino acid levels was completely abrogated by the concomitant treatment with N-acetylcysteine (107). The results showed the benefit of N-acetylcysteine was mainly seen in persons with lower than median plasma cysteine and asparagine concentrations. Persons with high postabsorptive plasma cysteine and asparagine levels showed a substantial exercise-induced increase in muscle functions, both with and without N-acetylcysteine treatment. On average, persons with low amino acid homeostasis did not benefit at all from the muscle exercise program unless they were supplemented with N-acetylcysteine. It was not possible to define a priori subgroups that would either need cysteine supplementation or not. Cysteine supplementation would have to be used by all to ensure exercise benefits for everybody. It should also be noted that the observed benefits for muscle function were obtained at a daily dose of 1.8 grams N-acetylcysteine, which was insufficient to detectably increase the fasted plasma cysteine and asparagine concentrations and amino acid homeostasis in the early morning. However, these results were derived from a single clinical study and need to be confirmed.

Incidentally, this study also revealed that the plasma level of the inflammatory cytokine tumor necrosis factor α (TNF-α) increased significantly during the exercise program and cysteine supplementation completely prevented this increase (152). Another study on healthy, young subjects showed a similar increase in TNF-α levels during physical exercise. In this case, this increase was prevented by cysteine supplementation in combination with antioxidant vitamins A, C, and E (363). The effects of cysteine supplementation on TNF-α concentrations are particularly relevant in view of the fact that some authors view aging as a process of chronic inflammation (45).

Physical exercise has been considered as a therapeutic tool to increase muscle mass and muscle function, but it was found to cause the oxidation of glutathione in the blood (309, 323). This oxidation was ameliorated by treatment with N-acetylcysteine (323). Five independent placebo-controlled clinical studies have shown furthermore that cysteine supplementation by N-acetylcysteine or a cysteine-rich whey protein caused a significant decrease in body fat (159, 190, 202, 82, 128). These findings deserve special attention because it is extremely difficult with any standard diet to maintain muscle mass without gaining weight and body fat or maintain a constant body weight without losing skeletal muscle mass. This effect of cysteine supplementation is again best explained by the redox sensitivity of the insulin receptor signaling cascade. The hepatic lipid metabolism is strongly regulated by the PPARγ coactivator-1, PGC-1α. PGC-1α is induced upon fasting (220, 384) and inhibited through phosphorylation by protein kinase Akt2 (PKBß), that is, by activation of the insulin receptor signaling cascade (218). Accordingly, PGC-1α (like autophagy) is mainly active in the postabsorptive state. As PGC-1α stimulates fatty acid ß-oxidation and shifts fuel usage from glucose to lipids (220), an aberrant increase in postabsorptive insulin receptor signaling activity provides a plausible explanation for the observed association between low postabsorptive plasma thiol levels and hyperlipidemia or obesity (107). Whereas, in the diabetic state, the liver is unresponsive to insulin with regard to the postprandial suppression of glucose output, it continues to produce large amounts of lipids, as expected from an aberrant activation of the insulin receptor signaling cascade (94, 98).

In several clinical studies, cysteine supplementation also yielded significant improvements in cardiovascular disease. In a placebo-controlled, double-blind trial of forty patients with peripheral artery disease, intravenous administration of glutathione improved macrocirculatory and microcirculatory parameters (14). In another study of sixteen patients, intracoronary infusion of N-acetylcysteine was found to augment acetylcholine-mediated microvascular dilation, indicating enhanced endothelial-dependent vasomotion. Incidentally, coronary vascular resistance was decreased, and coronary blood flow significantly increased (7). In patients with end-stage renal failure, N-acetylcysteine was shown to reduce cardiovascular events (346) and improve pulse pressure and endothelial function (313).

Significant effects of N-acetylcysteine on aging-related parameters have also been shown in several animal studies. Feeding of N-acetylcysteine-containing pellets to forty-eight-week-old mice for twenty-four weeks caused a significant decrease in protein oxidation in synaptic mitochondria of the brain in comparison with untreated control mice (21). Chronic dietary administration of N-acetylcysteine was also shown to preserve mitochondrial proteins involved in oxidative phosphorylation in the liver of senescent mice (251). Feeding of N-acetylcysteine-containing pellets to mice from twelve months until twenty-eight months (when they were killed) resulted in a significant increase in ATP-stimulated respiration in brain mitochondria. In addition, N-acetylcysteine treatment reversed the age-related decline in cytochrome C content and decrease in cytostolic glutathione in the brain (74).

With regard to age-related functional changes, N-acetylcysteine was found to ameliorate memory loss in rats (235). Again, this was associated with a reduced rate of protein oxidation and lipid peroxidation in brain synaptic mitochondria. Finally, N-acetylcysteine was shown to prevent accelerated atherosclerosis in an animal model (167).

Limits of cysteine supplementation

Whereas a daily dose of 1.8 grams N-acetylcysteine corresponding to 1.4 grams cysteine was found to significantly decrease the *basic* insulin responsiveness in the fasted state (159) and to increase skeletal muscle function in frail elderly patients (152), this dose failed in both of these studies to increase the amino acid homeostasis as indicated by the postabsorptive plasma cysteine and asparagine concentrations in the early morning. The attempt to restore the youthful state of the oxidative spiral of figure 5/figure 10 had obviously failed. It may therefore be tempting to consider higher doses of cysteine supplementation.

Glutathione biosynthesis proceeds up to a certain glutathione concentration where glutathione competes with glutamate for the glutamate binding site of glutamate cysteine ligase thereby causing the feedback inhibition of the first step in its own biosynthesis (243). Thereafter, any excess of cysteine is catabolized into various metabolic products, including sulfate and protons (78,231,144). One of the major adverse effects of excessive cysteine intake is the formation of large amounts of metabolic acid.

At doses of about 2 to 5 grams per day the cysteine derivative N-acetylcysteine was found to cause a significant increase in the plasma concentrations of amino acids including cystine (that is the oxidized form of cysteine), glutamine,and arginine in healthy volunteers (unpublished observation) and in patients with HIV infection (105,108). This is a potentially useful effect in certain diseases and conditions with abnormally low cystine and glutamine levels which include HIV infection, sepsis, major injury, trauma, cancer,Crohn's disease, ulcerative colitis,chronic fatigue syndrome, overtraining (105,108). Circumstantial evidence suggests that the abnormally low amino acid levels in these conditions and the increase in plasma amino acid levels after supplementation of high doses of cysteine, may be based, at least to some extent, on the formation of metabolic acid and the pH-dependent regulation of the hepatic urea production rate (105). Such a high dose of cysteine supplementation should therefore be adequately monitored and used with caution.

Daily doses of 1.8 grams N-acetylcysteine corresponding to 1.4 grams cysteine were found to decrease the *basic* insulin responsiveness without raising blood glucose levels beyond the normal level (159), but independent studies of volunteers after intensive physical exercise and elderly persons, i.e., two groups of persons with moderate insulin resistance, had shown that both groups had, on the average relatively high plasma amino acid concentrations including high cystine concentrations without a corresponding increase in the concentration of reduced cysteine (158).. Even a moderate insulin resitance may therefore bear the risk that any decrease in amino acid clearance causes a stronger increase in the plasma concentration of the oxidized relative to the reduced form of cysteine and accordingly an oxidative shift in the plasma redox status. Such a shift would alter the set points of redox-sensitive signaling pathways (102). Because the oxidized form cystine is twice as big as the reduced amino acid cysteine, cystine is not readily transported into cells and tissues (22) and is therefore accumulating in the plasma and as such not as readily available for intracellular glutathione biosynthesis as plasma cysteine.

A similar increase in plasma cystine without a corresponding increase in reduced cysteine was occasionally observed after continuous low dose cysteine supplementation. As creatine was previously found to reverse the decrease in insulin responsiveness by N-acetylcysteine in a placebo-controlled study (159), it was not surprising to see that the undesirable change in plasma cystine concentration and redox status was effectively prevented and even reversed by using cysteine in combination with creatine. This strategy is also being used in the guidelines described in addendum one.

Cysteine supplementation by cysteine-rich whey proteins has the additional advantage that whey stimulates insulin release and decreases the postprandial blood glucose concentration in both healthy persons and patients with type 2 diabetes. This effect is at least partly mediated by the constituent amino acids leucine, valine, lysine and isoleucine

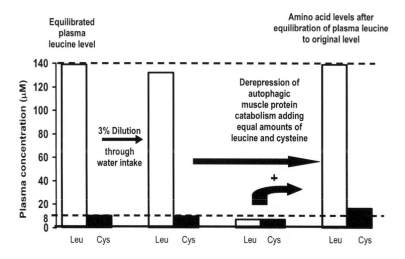

Fig. 12. *Water-assisted autophagy* (hypothetical example). The principle of *water-assisted autophagy* is illustrated by assuming a starting condition where the regulatory amino acid levels are in equilibrium, including plasma leucine at approximately one hundred and forty μM (see upper dotted line). This starting condition implies that protein catabolism is approximately zero and autophagy is largely suppressed. The plasma cysteine concentration is approximately eight μM (lower dotted line), which is typical for the elderly (figure 6). It is then assumed that these amino acids are diluted by 3 percent through oral water intake during the late night. This generates a temporary imbalance and decreases the leucine concentration to approximately one hundred and thirty-six μM, which, in turn, increases the probability of autophagy. This derepression of autophagic protein catabolism ends when the original, equilibrated plasma level of regulatory amino acids is reestablished (figure 3). As the skeletal muscle protein contains approximately similar amounts of cysteine and leucine, the temporary activation of autophagy leads to a similar absolute increase in the plasma concentration of both amino acids and accordingly to an overproportional relative increase in plasma cysteine concentration. In this example, both the plasma leucine and cysteine concentrations are increased by an absolute increment of approximately four μM, which brings the cysteine concentration to twelve μM, that is, the typical postabsorptive cysteine concentration of healthy young persons (figure 6). Even smaller incremental changes in regulatory amino acid concentrations would still lead to a large relative increase in plasma cysteine.

Water-assisted Autophagy: Targeting the Regulatory Amino Acids and the Target of Rapamycin

The term *water-assisted autophagy* is proposed to describe a method to enhance the postabsorptive autophagic protein catabolism through additional water intake during the late night. According to the principal mechanism of amino acid homeostasis (figure 3), an incremental dilution of the blood plasma and corresponding incremental decrease in the plasma concentrations of leucine and other regulatory amino acids is expected to derepress autophagy up to the point where the original equilibrium of regulatory amino acids is reestablished. This process is expected to increase the plasma cysteine concentration, thereby facilitating the biosynthesis of glutathione (figure 12). In the example of figure 12, the amino acids are diluted by 3.3 percent and the plasma concentration of the regulatory amino acid leucine is accordingly decreased from its equilibrium at 140 μM down to 135.8 μM. This may temporarily derepress the autophagic activity until the plasma leucine concentration again reaches its original equilibrium of one hundred and forty μM. As the cysteine and leucine content of muscle protein is in the same order of magnitude, this autophagy-mediated increase in plasma leucine by 4.2 mM will be accompanied by a similar increase in plasma cysteine by approximately 4 mM. This implies the originally small concentration of approximately 8 μM plasma cysteine, which is typical for the elderly, will increase by 50 percent to a level typical for young, healthy persons (figure 6). This strategy is therefore expected to support glutathione biosynthesis during times of starvation and decrease the oxidative stress that would otherwise result from the low postabsorptive plasma cysteine and intracellular glutathione levels. The method of *water-assisted autophagy* remains to be studied more systematically. In addition, elderly people are encouraged to drink more than needed during the day to satisfy their thirst. Because elderly often show a reduced sensation of thirst, many elderly do not drink enough to support optimal cellular functions. It has been estimated that a daily water intake of 3.7 liters for adult men and 2.7 liters for adult women meets the need of the vast majority of persons (310).

Chapter Six

Dietary Components with Effects on the Cycle

Optimizing the Dietary Carbohydrate Intake

Being a process of self-eating, autophagy needs to be limited in time and balanced by a period of strong protein synthesis. As the insulin signaling mechanism suppresses autophagy, the nightly period of autophagic activity is normally terminated by the daily intake of carbohydrate, which induces the production of insulin. This is often, but not always, accompanied by the consumption of dietary protein as a source of amino acids, which further downregulate autophagy.

In addition, the daily consumption of carbohydrate provides an optimal source of energy for the brain. The human brain works best with glucose, and an adequate dietary carbohydrate intake is required to avoid a state of low plasma glucose levels called *hypoglycemia*. If plasma glucose levels decline, glucose levels are reestablished through the induction of hypoglycemic response factors, such as cortisol, glucagon, and adrenaline. Among other consequences, these factors trigger the release of amino acids from skeletal muscle protein in a process unrelated to autophagy. The production of hypoglycemic response factors should be reserved for emergency situations only. One of the important quasi-pharmacological effects of the dietary carbohydrate intake is to prevent conditions of hypoglycemia. This is one of the reasons to avoid extreme calorie restriction. To avoid any hypoglycemic response during the day while practicing moderate calorie restriction, it is recommended to consume moderate amounts of carbohydrate frequently in relatively short time intervals throughout the day (figure 13). This is essentially the same recommendation that is typically given to diabetic patients. Any excess of dietary carbohydrate intake is a risk factor for the development of obesity and diabetes.

Creatine, Methionine and Arginine

Creatine is a nutritional supplement that is frequently sold in fitness clubs. Bodybuilders consume rather high amounts (up to twenty grams per day). But it is less well-known that creatine is a normal constituent of our diet and contained in substantial quantities in meat (animal muscle) and chicken soup (muscle extract). The skeletal muscle tissues of a healthy man of 75kg may contain more than 70g of creatine or creatine phosphate, and additional amounts of creatine are contained in the nervous tissues. In the context of the aging process and life span extension, it is important to note that a high dietary intake of creatine is likely to increase the insulin signaling activity, which then compromises autophagy and cysteine homeostasis. Creatine supplementation was shown to reverse the effect of cysteine supplementation on the basal (postabsorptive) insulin responsiveness, which has been described previously.

Methionine, glycine, and arginine are required not only as amino acid precursors for protein synthesis but also for the biosynthesis of creatine. Because creatine is one of the quantitatively most important methylated metabolites and guanido-derivatives in the body, a diet low in methionine or arginine containing proteins may limit the availability of creatine in muscle and brain tissues. Conversely, creatine supplementation may have a sparing effect on the free methionine and arginine pools.

However, creatine deficiency states with consequences for the central nervous system and muscle tissues have also been occasionally reported. The human body can synthesize creatine, but the quantity is not always sufficient to satisfy the needs. According to published data on the mean urinary excretion of creatinine, adult men convert approximately 1.8g and women 1.2g of creatine into creatinine each day and would have to replace this either through dietary creatine

Fig. 13

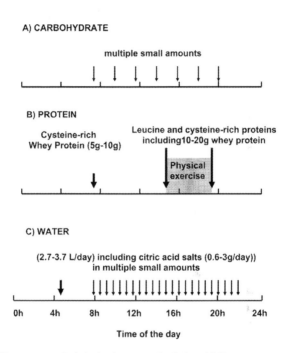

Fig. 13. Recommended daily dietary schedules. A) It is recommended to consume moderate amounts of carbohydrates frequently in relatively short time intervals throughout the day. B) To account for the relatively low cysteine and glutathione concentrations in the postabsorptive state, it is recommended to eat five to ten grams of cysteine-rich whey protein early in the morning. In addition, ten to thirty grams of cysteine- and leucine-rich whey protein should ideally be consumed immediately before and/or after a bout of physical exercise. The rest of the daily dietary protein intake up to a total amount slightly larger than the recommended dietary allowance (RDA) of 0.8 grams per kilogram of body weight may be distributed over the day to minimize the breakdown of protein during the day. C) To enhance the autophagic activity in the early morning hours, it is recommended to drink one hundred to five hundred milliliters of water two to three hours before breakfast. In addition, it is recommended to drink water frequently during the day in a total amount of 2.7 to 3.7 liters per day. These amounts of water may contain a total of 0.6 to 3.0 grams of citric acid salts per day to compensate for the net acid load (chapter 7).

intake or through biosynthesis from the three precurcor amino acids which involves a substantial demand on these amino acids. It is therefore reasonable to consume moderate amounts of dietary creatine. Persons who follow their body weight closely on a daily basis often find that they gain weight if they take creatine and lose weight if they stop taking it. In these cases, the body weight can be used as a guideline, and the creatine consumption should be adjusted to an intermediate level. At higher doses of cysteine supplementation (see addendum one) it is recommended to use creatine in one of three alternating periods as a tool to modify the effect of cysteine supplementation on insulin responsiveness.

Dietary Magnesium Intake

Like cysteine and creatine, magnesium is a normal component of our daily diet that happens to have a significant impact on the insulin signaling mechanism. A diet high in magnesium is therefore expected to have a negative effect on autophagy, cysteine homeostasis, and, ultimately, oxidative stress. But it is not advisable to deliberately limit the dietary intake of magnesium because magnesium is a required cofactor for over three hundred enzyme systems. One may therefore want to follow the (RDA) of four hundred and twenty milligrams per day for men and three hundred and twenty milligrams per day for women. The use of magnesium supplements is strongly recommended during periods of dietary restriction.

Scientific Evidence

The optimal strategy for dietary carbohydrate intake

As the loss of body cell mass and risk of hypoglycemic episodes are the major adverse effects of calorie restriction, it is recommended to restrict the intake of dietary carbohydrate only to the point where a constant body cell mass can be maintained over long periods and hypoglycemic episodes are being kept to a minimum. Hypoglycemic hormones have a relatively long life span in the blood, and the skeletal muscle catabolism may continue even when dietary glucose has become available again. To avoid any hypoglycemic response during the day, it may be advantageous to distribute the carbohydrate intake evenly throughout the day. It is recommended to consume moderate amounts of carbohydrates every two hours during the day (figure 13). A similar recommendation is typically given to diabetic patients.

Dietary intake of creatine, methionine and arginine

The rate of phosphorylation of target proteins by the insulin receptor kinase is determined, at least to some extent, by the availability of ATP as a key substrate and the removal of ADP as its product. Creatine

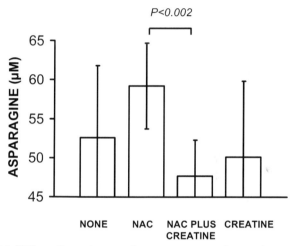

Fig. 14. Effect of cysteine supplementation together, with or without creatine, on the postabsorptive plasma asparagine level (μM$\pm$S.D). A simple way of testing the effect of creatine on the postabsorptive amino acid homeostasis is illustrated by this anecdotal example. A sixty-year-old male volunteer used the indicated supplements, N-acetylcysteine (NAC), creatine, or NAC plus creatine during consecutive periods each lasting approximately eight to twelve weeks. Postabsorptive plasma amino acid levels were determined four to six times during each of these periods. The figure shows the mean plasma asparagine levels ($\pm$S.D). The data shows the plasma asparagine levels during periods with NAC plus creatine were significantly lower than during the period with NAC alone (W. Dröge, unpublished observation).

phosphate, in combination with the enzyme creatine kinase, converts ADP into ATP, and the concentration of creatine phosphate thereby facilitates the insulin signaling activity in the skeletal muscle tissue. In line with these biochemical mechanisms, even small doses of creatine were shown to reverse the downregulation of the basal (postabsorptive) insulin responsiveness by cysteine supplementation (159), suggesting dietary creatine may also have a negative effect on autophagy and amino acid homeostasis and should be used with caution. To test this prediction, the effects of creatine intake on the amino acid homeostasis have been determined by measuring the postabsorptive plasma asparagine levels in a small pilot study. The anecdotal observations in figure 14 show the asparagine concentrations were indeed significantly decreased after cysteine supplementation in combination with creatine, as compared to cysteine supplementation alone.

This potentially negative effect of creatine consumption has to be balanced with the positive functions of creatine. Creatine is a natural constituent of skeletal muscle and brain tissues, and it plays an important role in the energy metabolism of these tissues (341,116, 340, 20, 154, 389, 164). Muscle tissue may contain more than thirty mM creatine phosphate. Considering that muscle mass accounts for almost half of our body weight, creatine is one of the quantitatively most important metabolites in our body. The endogenous capacity to synthesize creatine within our body is not always sufficient to satisfy the needs (49). The biosynthesis of creatine involves the methylation of its biosynthetic precursor guanidoacetate which is derived from arginine and glycine. As methylation requires methionine, a protein diet with sufficient methionine and arginine is needed for adequate creatine biosynthesis. Several authors have described pathological consequences of creatine deficient states of the central nervous system (341, 116, 340) and muscle tissues (20).

Athletes have extensively used creatine monohydrate in doses of up to twenty grams per day to increase their muscle mass. Several studies in both elderly and young adults have shown that the effect of resistance exercise on strength and muscle mass and/or fiber size can be enhanced by creatine supplementation (43, 48, 49, 82, 161, 71). It has also been found that the maintenance of muscle mass in older women is correlated with a relatively high intake of protein from animal sources (224), which, compared to other protein sources, is particularly high in creatine. Beef, like many other forms of muscle tissues, contains approximately five grams of creatine per kilogram. However, as the intervention studies have been performed over periods of six to fourteen weeks, there is little information about possible adverse effects of creatine supplementation over many months or years. In view of all these different aspects, creatine-containing diets should be used in a carefully balanced way.

Dietary magnesium intake

Together with cysteine and creatine, magnesium is the third major dietary component with a significant impact on the insulin receptor signaling cascade. Being a protein tyrosine kinase, the insulin receptor requires the MgATP complex as a cosubstrate in protein phosphorylation (163). In line with this requirement for magnesium, it was found that the decreased insulin responsiveness in patients with type 2 diabetes is frequently associated with abnormally low plasma magnesium concentrations (286, 29, 368) and magnesium supplementation increases insulin responsiveness and/or glucose disposal (284, 261, 299).

Although the effect of magnesium supplementation on the autophagic activity has not been systemically studied, it may be wise to avoid excessive doses of magnesium supplements. However, as the magnesium ATP complex is critically required by all cells and in multiple biochemical processes, magnesium deprivation is not the method of choice to downregulate the postabsorptive (basic) insulin receptor signaling activity. The RDA is four hundred and twenty milligrams per day for men and three hundred and twenty milligrams per day for women (337).

Chapter Seven

Complementary Strategies to Optimize the
Interventions

The Health Hazard of Metabolic Acidification

The negative aspects of acidic conditions in food, biological fluids, or tissues are widely known. If milk has turned sour, it contains acid and does not taste good. If the salad contains too much vinegar, it is too acidic. Again, it tastes bad. If certain forms of air pollution lead to acid rain, this is harmful for trees and eventually can devastate whole forests. If an athlete runs two hundred meters at maximum speed, his muscles get sour (acidic) and do not function well until they have recovered their normal acid-base balance or acid-alkali balance, as it is also called. Too much base (or alkali) is not good for our tissues either. Our cells, tissues, and body fluids need to be well-balanced. They should be neutral.

The proper acid-base balance is achieved through an adequate balance of food types. Ideally, our diet should include 75 to 85 percent alkali-producing foods and 15 to 25 percent acid-producing foods. Alkali-producing foods include grains, most fruits, and vegetables. Protein-rich food such as meat, fish, dairy, and egg whites are the most important acid-producing foods.

There is now an increasing awareness that most people in North America are slightly but demonstrably acidic because the typical Western diet is overabundant in acid-producing foods. An easily demonstrable manifestation is the acidic urine. Although the body has built-in regulators (buffers) for regulating the internal acid-base balance, getting rid of excess acid comes at a price. The capacity to eliminate the acid through the kidneys is rather limited, and acid excretion is a burden to the kidneys. The ability of our blood to buffer the acid using its bicarbonate content is also extremely limited and compromises our ability to transport carbon dioxide, which we exhale. Eventually, most of the burden of buffering excess acid rests upon our bones at the expense of bone minerals. The best investigated and eventually most harmful consequence of the acidification of our body is the loss of bone mineral density, which can ultimately lead to the devastating disease of osteoporosis. While this is only one conspicuous and well-investigated example, the loss of optimal acid-based balance eventually compromises important functions in all cells and tissues in the body.

Increasing the dietary intake of cysteine increases the formation of metabolic acid in the tissues. It is therefore appropriate to combine the recommendation of cysteine supplementation with specific recommendations that can help to ameliorate the metabolic acidification.

In view of the mechanisms described in the first chapters, the problem of acidification should not be solved by simply reducing the consumption of cysteine-rich proteins. A better strategy would be to increase the consumption of dietary plant foods, such as leafy green vegetables, stalks, roots, and fruits that are metabolized into products that neutralize the acid. Ideally, the amounts of these plant foods should be sufficient to render the urine approximately neutral, that is, to adjust its pH to about 6.5 to 6.8. As such a drastic change in the habit of food consumption would be expected to increase the intake of carbohydrates and is unlikely to happen, supplementation of potassium and calcium salts of metabolizable organic acids or bicarbonate is an attractive alternative and becoming increasingly important. Also in this case, the amount should be adjusted to bring the urine pH to a value of 6.5 to 6.8. There is a convincing body of evidence that this strategy can decrease net acid production and enhance net calcium retention.

The Loss of Bone Mineral Density and Risk of Osteoporosis

Age-related bone loss is found in man and even more frequently in women. Although bone loss starts already in the third decade of life, it is most prevalent among postmenopausal women above the age of fifty. It is associated with an increased risk of bone fractures, notably hip fractures, and an increased probability of death in the year after fracture.

Strong clinical evidence shows that metabolic acidification leads to a loss of bone mineral density and is a risk factor for the development of osteoporosis. Dietary supplements of citric acid salts, such as potassium citrate and calcium citrate, decrease bone resorption and urinary calcium excretion. Calcium citrate was shown to increase bone mineral density. Within the tissues, citric acid salts are converted into bicarbonate. They have a strong effect on the acid-base balance and neutralize the metabolic acid generated from cysteine. The best clinical evidence was obtained with potassium citrate and calcium citrate, but sodium citrate, magnesium citrate, or the corresponding lactate salts can reasonably be expected to be as effective.

Comparison of Citric Acid Salts with Bicarbonate Salts

Bicarbonate salts are presently the most popular remedies against the health hazards of acidification. Many of the laboratory studies on the effects of acidification have been performed with bicarbonate rather than citrate salts, and various doses of bicarbonate were shown to increase the plasma bicarbonate concentration as a sign of decreased acidification. The consumption of bicarbonate salts has the disadvantage, however, that bicarbonate salts are converted in the stomach into chloride salts plus carbon dioxide. Citrate salts appear to be the more suitable agents to increase the bicarbonate concentration in the blood.

As the consumption of potassium citrate supplements reduces urinary calcium excretion, it also reduces the risk of kidney stones. Several clinical studies have shown that treatment with potassium citrate reduces the recurrence rate in patients with calcium stone disease.

Muscle Wasting as Another Consequence of Low-grade Metabolic Acidosis

The loss of bone mineral density is the best-investigated health hazard of metabolic acidosis, but not the only adverse effect. Several laboratories have shown that metabolic acidification also leads to the degradation of skeletal muscle protein and loss of lean body mass.

Dietary Proteins and Physical Exercise to Maintain Skeletal Muscle Function

As old cities are rejuvenated by removing old and damaged structures and building new and modern structures in their place, a healthy body also replaces damaged parts by new ones. Specifically, young, healthy persons are capable of compensating the process of autophagic protein breakdown by a corresponding process of protein synthesis during daytime.

Although autophagy appears to be the more important life span-determining factor, the maintenance of the protein mass and, notably, the skeletal muscle mass in the course of aging is presently one of the most difficult issues in aging research. The difficulty of maintaining an adequate balance between protein breakdown and protein synthesis is exemplified by the massive loss of muscle mass, a process called sarcopenia that starts in the fourth decade of life and accelerates in old age. As the loss of muscle mass is associated with a loss of muscle function, it increases the risk of falls and fractures, compromises the ability to visit friends or maintain other social functions, and contributes to the loss of quality of life in old age.

As skeletal muscle tissues represent about half of the protein mass in the human body, the loss of muscle mass means a net loss of protein. The factors that determine the rate of protein synthesis in old age have been studied intensively in recent years by several laboratories. As dietary proteins provide the amino acids needed for protein synthesis (figure 15), inadequate protein consumption inevitably leads to a loss of protein and contributes frequently to the development of sarcopenia. The RDA for both men and women is 0.8 grams of good quality protein per kilogram of body weight per day, but this recommendation has been criticized as being insufficient on the basis of methodological considerations. And even the recommendation to increase the dietary protein intake would not generally prevent the loss of muscle and protein mass in old age. The mechanism of sarcopenia is not well understood, and a treatment that reverses this process has not yet been reported. The best available strategies to optimize skeletal muscle protein synthesis as well as muscle mass and muscle function in old age involve a combination of dietary protein supplements and physical exercise. They will be discussed subsequently.

Regulation of Protein Synthesis by Amino Acids

Skeletal muscle protein synthesis is strongly stimulated by amino acids and insulin through the same signaling pathway that downregulates autophagy (figure 3). *This signaling pathway is inhibited by rapamycin (see chapter 5).* A small group of amino acids called regulatory amino acids, such as leucine, has been identified as the most effective stimulators of protein synthesis and inhibitors of autophagy. Muscle protein synthesis in both young and elderly people is increased by feeding either mixed amino acids or proteins. In this context, the cysteine- and leucine-rich whey proteins were found to be markedly more effective than casein.

Potentially Adverse Effects of a High Dietary Protein Intake

It is generally recommended that the daily protein consumption should not comprise more than 30 percent of the total energy intake, but the Tolerable Upper Intake Level (UL) for protein or specific amino acids and potentially adverse effects have not been systematically investigated. Certain specific points, however, should be addressed here.

- It is known that the most common dietary protein sources typically have a high fat content. This problem ought to be minimized by focusing on low-fat proteins.

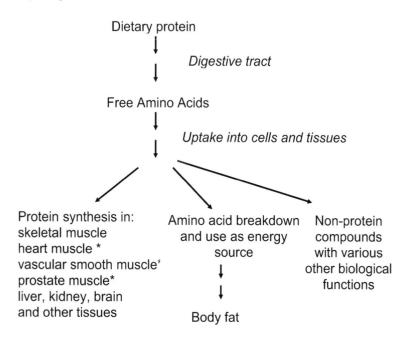

Fig. 15. Utilization of dietary proteins (simplified illustration). In the digestive tract, proteins are broken down into their constituent amino acids, which are then transported into the blood and then moved into the cells and tissues. The resulting synthesis of host proteins facilitates the hypertrophy of skeletal muscle tissue, which is generally desirable as well as in heart muscle, vascular smooth muscle cells, and prostate muscle, where hypertrophy is generally undesirable.

Another portion of amino acids is used as a source of energy, and some of the amino acids are converted into non-protein compounds with various other biological functions. The conversion of amino acids into glucose and indirectly into body fat is largely determined by the free amino acid concentration and its persistence over time. Skeletal muscle protein synthesis is faster in young than in elderly persons. It is also faster after physical exercise than during sedentary periods. The more rapid clearance of amino acids into the skeletal muscle in young adults and after physical exercise renders amino acids less available for undesirable protein synthesis activities in other tissues or conversion into body fat.

- The undesirable formation of metabolic acid from sulfur-con-taining proteins should be compensated by a high intake of fruits and vegetables or potassium citrate supplements, as described previously.

- A potentially adverse effect of a high protein intake is that a relatively high proportion of ingested amino acids is converted into glucose and indirectly into body fat (figure 15). This problem would have to be compensated by a decreased consumption of fat.

- A somewhat greater challenge is that we know little about the effects of the dietary protein consumption on the undesirable hypertrophy of tissues other than skeletal muscle, such as the heart, prostate, vascular smooth muscle cells, and so on (figure 15). The weight of the heart increases with age, compromising its functional capacity. Vascular smooth muscle cells around the arteries play an important role in the differential regulation of blood flow to different parts of the body. Age-related changes, such as smooth muscle cell proliferation and hyperplasia, potentially contribute to the thickening and stiffening of the arterial walls. The putative effects of dietary protein intake on these types of undesirable hypertrophic processes have not yet been systematically investigated, but they are likely to play a quite significant role in the age-related decline. Therefore, one would like to have a method that selectively enhances the anabolic effects of dietary protein consumption on skeletal muscle tissues while avoiding undesirable hypertrophic processes in other tissues.

The Importance of Muscular Activity and Benefits from Physical Exercise

Physical exercise is extremely important in this context for several reasons. Regular physical exercise is the only known method to extend the average life span in humans, at least in statistical terms. Resistance training is the best-investigated method shown to increase muscle mass and muscle function, even in elderly persons. In view of the role of the autophagic protein catabolism during the night as a life span-determining factor and the need to compensate the autophagy-mediated loss of protein mass by a corresponding amount of protein synthesis during daytime, it is important to note that both resistance exercise and endurance exercise stimulate preferentially the synthesis of skeletal muscle protein. Physical exercise may be the best available method to direct the utilization of dietary amino acids preferentially into skeletal muscle protein synthesis at the expense of undesirable hypertrophic processes, but this reasonable assumption remains to be confirmed.

Effects of Protein Intake Together with Resistance Exercise on Muscle Function

Expectedly, the stimulation of muscle protein synthesis by exercise is markedly enhanced if exercise is combined with amino acids or protein supplements. The best effects were generally obtained when amino acids were given shortly after exercise. Again, whey protein was found to be more effective than casein or soy protein if given after exercise.

Although dietary protein or amino acid intake consistently enhances muscle protein synthesis in the context of resistance exercise, protein or amino acid supplements often failed to further enhance muscle functions beyond the effect of physical exercise alone, except in certain circumstances that need to be discussed here. One of the most important findings was that the effect of physical exercise on muscle mass and muscle function was significantly enhanced if whey protein was given immediately before and after exercise, but not if the same daily dose was given in the morning and late evening. Whey protein was shown to be more effective than casein, especially in the elderly.

In contrast to casein, whey protein passes rather quickly through the digestive tract and leads to a rapid and high rise in amino acid concentrations in the blood within about two hours. These high amino acid concentrations enhance skeletal muscle protein synthesis in both the young and elderly, but would also cause a relatively high rate of amino acid breakdown and undesirable protein synthesis in certain hypertrophic tissues unless rapidly cleared from the blood by the skeletal muscle tissue. By stimulating skeletal muscle protein synthesis, physical exercise is the best method to facilitate this process, provided the increase in amino acid concentration coincides with the muscle protein synthesis that follows the exercise. As a crude guideline, it is recommended to consume dietary whey protein immediately before or after exercise at daily amounts of approximately ten to thirty grams, depending on body weight and exercise intensity.

A regular intake of whey protein according to this schedule has three advantages compared to other proteins:

1. The relatively brief, but high, peaks of amino acid concentrations and notably the high leucine concentration provide a strong anabolic stimulus, especially in the elderly.

2. By consuming whey protein immediately before and/or after physical exercise, the amino acids are delivered preferentially to the skeletal muscle tissues and not to other tissues that would respond with undesirable hypertrophy.

3. The regular use of the cysteine-rich whey protein at the indicated daily dose is an ideal method of cysteine supplementation that can be reasonably expected to ameliorate the oxidative stress resulting from the oxidative spiral in figure 5/figure 10. The rest of the daily dietary protein intake, including various slow proteins, may be distributed throughout the day to minimize an undesirable protein breakdown during daytime. The total protein consumption may be slightly above the daily RDA of 0.8 grams per kilogram of body weight, depending on the level of physical activity.

Scientific Evidence

Metabolic acidification and loss of bone mineral density

There is an increasing awareness of the health hazards caused by the diet's net acid load and resulting metabolic acidification (80, 123, 124). It has been shown that low-grade metabolic acidosis is quite common and increases with age and contributes to the age-related loss of bone and skeletal muscle mass (123, 124). A major cause of the chronic low-grade metabolic acidosis is the relatively large proportion of dietary foods, notably cysteine-rich proteins, whose metabolism yields non-carbonic acids, such as sulfuric acid, combined with an insufficient proportion of foods whose metabolism yields alkali bicarbonate (212, 201). Clinical studies indicate that protein-rich diet causes an increase in acid load to the body, leading to increased acid excretion (42, 314).

Using carefully controlled conditions, several clinical studies have indicated that acid loads (as generated by dietary protein or ammonium chloride) cause an increase in urinary calcium excretion without a change in intestinal calcium absorption, indicating a decrease in net calcium retention (208, 209). Similar effects have been shown in patients with osteoporosis. In line with these findings, persistent chronic metabolic acidosis has been suggested as a cause of osteoporosis (26, 207).

Osteoporosis and generally accepted surrogate parameters

Age-related bone loss is found mainly in women but frequently also in men. Cross-sectional data suggest that bone loss begins between the ages of eighteen and thirty years, but the process is slow (320). A recent analysis revealed that, among postmenopausal women aged fifty years or more, 7.2 percent have osteoporosis and 36 percent have osteopenia (329). The lifetime risk for fragility fractures due to osteoporosis after the age of fifty years is about 50 percent in women and 20 percent in men (86). Osteoporotic hip fractures are associated with a 20 percent excess mortality in the year after fracture (262). According to the World Health Organization (WHO) criteria, osteoporosis is commonly diagnosed based on the patient's bone mineral density (BMD) compared with the average peak BMD of young adult women (172, 176, 171).

Citric acid salts of alkali and earth alkali to prevent loss of bone mineral density

In a crossover study involving eighteen postmenopausal women at the Center for Mineral Metabolism and Clinical Research in Texas, it was shown that the combined treatment with potassium citrate (4.3 grams per day) and calcium citrate (eight hundred milligrams per day) inhibited bone resorption, increased absorbed calcium, and decreased urinary calcium excretion (1). No adverse effects have been reported. The same research group also reported a study involving sixteen men and five women with kidney stones showing that treatment with potassium citrate (2.2 to 6.6 grams per day) from eleven to one hundred and twenty months caused a significant increase in BMD and a corresponding increase in urinary pH up to 6.7 (279). This study did not include a control group not receiving potassium citrate treatment, but it had a historical control. In another study of sixty postmenopausal women at the University of California, San Francisco, it was found that the addition of oral potassium citrate (9.7 grams per day) to a high salt diet prevented the increase in urine calcium excretion and bone resorption caused by high salt intake (322). Again, no adverse effects have been reported. Dawson-Hughes and Harris (91) have shown in a placebo-controlled trial of three hundred and forty-two healthy elderly men and women over a three-year period that a supplement of calcium salts of metabolizable organic acids, including citrate, caused a significant increase in total body and femoral neck bone mineral density only in subjects with the highest tertile of protein intake. Conversely, the high protein intake had a positive effect on BMD if (and only if) combined with the supplement (91). Marangella and others (233) reported a nonrandomized, unblinded study on postmenopausal women showing that treatment with potassium citrate (four to seven grams per day) over a three-month period caused a significant improvement of several surrogate markers of bone resorption and an increase in urinary pH up to 6.3. Again, no adverse effects have been reported (233). In view of the health burden of osteoporosis, these findings from several independent research centers provide an opportunity to reduce an important health risk.

Although the best clinical evidence was obtained with potassium citrate alone or in combination with calcium citrate, supportive evidence suggests that other alkaline and earth alkali citrates are as effective and combinations of potassium citrate with calcium citrate plus moderate amounts of magnesium citrate may even be advantageous.

As citric acid is a metabolizable organic acid and leads to the formation of bicarbonate in cells and tissues, potassium citrate is well-suited to neutralize the metabolic acid generated by cysteine supplementation (figure 16). The strong effect of alkaline citrate on the acid-base balance indirectly affects the urine pH and citrate excretion (206, 146). Citrate excretion is decreased when acid excretion increases (2, 369) and rises when acid production and net acid excretion decreases, as during the administration of potassium bicarbonate (210) or potassium citrate (283). Urinary citrate excretion decreases by about 0.02 millimoles per day for each milliequivalent per day increment in urinary net acid excretion. Conversely, citrate excretion increases by an equivalent amount as net acid excretion decreases (210, 207, 42). In addition, alkaline salts of metabolizable organic anions were shown to decrease the efflux of calcium from bone, thereby decreasing the urinary calcium secretion as described subsequently.

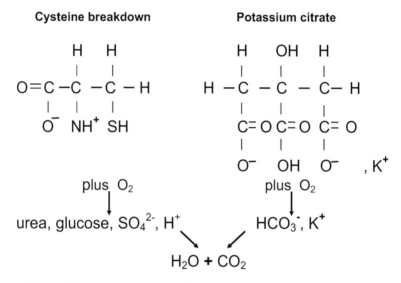

Fig. 16. Potassium citrate complementing cysteine supplementation. During cysteine breakdown, the sulfhydryl group is oxidized and ultimately yields sulfate and protons (H+). This acid load can cause a number of health problems unless neutralized. The dietary potassium citrate supplement is converted by the citric acid cycle in cells and tissues into potassium and hydrogen carbonate (HCO3-). Ultimately, the hydrogen carbonate anions neutralize the protons to yield carbon dioxide and water.

Effect of acid-base equilibrium on bone density (buffering of acid and base by bones)

The following summarizes mechanistic studies indicating that citrate supplements have a direct effect on BMD by decreasing the calcium efflux from bone. Protein-derived metabolic acids are buffered to some extent by bicarbonate, thereby causing a moderate decrease in plasma bicarbonate concentration (metabolic acidosis) and decrease in urinary pH (50). In addition, metabolic acid formation is buffered by bone tissue in a process involving the release of calcium from bone mineral (318, 51, 211, 54). When acid production was experimentally increased among healthy subjects, renal acid excretion was not increased as much as acid production so acid balances became positive because of bone buffering of retained H^+ and loss of calcium from bone into the urine (211). In vitro studies from several laboratories consistently showed that metabolic acidosis increases net calcium efflux from the bone (54, 13, 136, 290, 50, 54, 65, 198, 336). The calcium efflux is the consequence of the dissolution of bone mineral associated with an increase in osteoclastic bone resorption and decrease in osteoblastic bone formation (50, 52, 53, 198, 336, 6). Even at a constant pH, a decrease in bicarbonate concentration was found to cause a marked increase in calcium efflux (52).

Another mechanism implicated in the effect of endogenous acid production on urinary calcium excretion is the linkage between urinary pH and renal tubular resorption of calcium (reviewed in 207).

The use of alkaline citrate rather than bicarbonate salts

Many of the in vivo studies cited previously have been performed with bicarbonate rather than citrate salts. Oral doses of potassium bicarbonate, for example, were shown to neutralize the endogenous acid production and increase the plasma bicarbonate concentration (318).

Administration of potassium or sodium bicarbonate to volunteers on animal protein diets was also shown to decrease urinary calcium excretion and enhance net calcium retention (226, 318, 127). However, as bicarbonate salts are largely neutralized by the hydrochloric acid content in the stomach (and vice versa), they are not the most suitable agents to increase the concentration of sodium bicarbonate in the blood. Sodium or potassium citrate salts have the advantage that they pass through the stomach and are taken up by cells and tissues, where they are ultimately metabolized to yield bicarbonate through the citric acid cycle (143).

Determining which mineral cation should be used

As fruits and vegetables contain considerable amounts of potassium salts of organic acids, potassium citrate may resemble the natural situation more closely than other citrate salts. In addition, the arterial sodium concentration affects the retention of water by the kidney (143). Lower sodium and high potassium intakes are associated with the reduction of hypertension (324). Most people do not generally achieve the required dietary intake of potassium (about 4.5 grams per day). However, as important signaling pathways in the vascular endothelium and carotid chemoreceptor are controlled by potassium ion channels (379, 327, 199), small changes in the arterial potassium ion concentration may have profound effects on the vascular tone, blood flow, and ventilation (191). In rare occasions, hyperkalemia was shown to cause a significant disturbance of cardiac function (160).

The question if sodium bicarbonate can substitute for potassium bicarbonate as a means to improve calcium balance has been a controversial issue (226, 210). The addition of potassium citrate to a diet high in sodium chloride was shown to prevent the increase in calcium loss and bone turnover markers caused by a high dietary salt intake alone in postmenopausal women (322). In another study on postmenopausal women, it was found that urinary calcium excretion was significantly decreased by treatment with potassium citrate alone. However, the treatment with potassium citrate in combination with calcium citrate was even more effective in inhibiting bone resorption and increasing absorbed calcium (305).

Effects of alkali and earth alkali citrates on the risk of kidney stones

To decrease the risk of bone fractures, it is generally recommended that persons at risk of fractures, notably postmenopausal women, increase their daily calcium intake and facilitate the calcium uptake by additional supplements of vitamin D (168). It was noted, however, that the most common type of calcium supplementation, that is, calcium carbonate supplementation, increases the risk of kidney stones (168), although one prospective cohort study revealed an inverse correlation between dietary calcium intake and risk of kidney stones (87). (See also women's health initiative (WHI) trial of calcium with vitamin D.) The majority of kidney stones are composed of calcium oxalate and/or apatite. A high urinary calcium excretion rate is a recognized risk factor for stone formation (205, 253, 6).

Increasing the dietary intake of potassium or supplementation of potassium bicarbonate or citrate was shown to reduce urinary calcium excretion (87, 270, 207) and reduce the risk of kidney stones (87). Potassium citrate is currently being used for the management of renal tubular acidosis with calcium stones, hypocitraturic calcium oxalate nephrolithiasis of any etiology, and uric acid lithiasis, with or without calcium stones. In two studies on the recurrence rate of calcium stone formers during treatment with alkaline citrate (23, 113) and one study on the clearance of stone fragments from the kidney (72), it has been shown that alkali citrate is effective in reducing the recurrence rate in patients with calcium stone disease. The doses were generally in the range between four to eight grams per day. In one case, they were shown to increase the urine pH to 6.3 (112). In the summary of the Consensus Conference on behalf of the Advisory Board of European Urilithiasis Research (354), it has been suggested that alkaline citrate might be most useful for patients with hypocitraturia, but its indication may be extended to all calcium stone formers, irrespective of urinary findings. Mild side effects were recorded in 42 percent of the treated patients, moderate in 26 percent, and severe (usually diarrhea) in 12 percent (354). It should be noted that the alkaline citrate salts were apparently not neutralized in these studies, for example, by additional free citric acid. This may leave room for improvement. The formation of clinically important calcium oxalate stones was shown to be inhibited by alkali citrate at physiological concentrations (135, 155). Citrate is capable of complexing with urinary calcium, thereby reducing the availability of calcium to crystallize as calcium oxalate, brushite, and apatite (206, 146).

By increasing the urine pH (206, 146), alkaline salts of metabolizable organic anions such as citrate also decrease the risk of uric acid stones (278, 234, 156). Uric acid is a weak organic acid with very low pH-dependent solubility in aqueous solutions (reviewed in 156).

Opposing effects of dietary protein intake on bone health (risk of osteoporosis)

In view of the role of the dietary net acid load on bone calcium homeostasis and impact of dietary protein on the net acid load, it may be assumed that decreasing dietary protein may be beneficial for bone health. However, an adequate supply of dietary protein was shown to be absolutely crucial for the maintenance of body cell mass and numerous cellular functions, including bone health. A study by Kerstetter and colleagues on healthy women (184) revealed that a protein intake of 0.7 grams per kilogram of body weight per day (slightly below the RDA of 0.8 grams per kilogram of body weight per day) led to impaired intestinal calcium absorption, whereas subjects consuming 1.0 gram per kilogram of body weight per day demonstrated little change in calcium homeostasis (reviewed in 210, 184). A more recent study revealed that increasing the protein diet from 1.0 to 2.1 grams per kilogram of body weight per day caused a dramatic increase in calcium absorption (185). A report on dietary intake data and corresponding proximal forearm bone variables determined by quantitative computer tomography in two hundred and twenty-nine healthy children and adolescents over a four-year period revealed a positive correlation between protein intake and bone variables, including bone cortex area and bone mineral content, and a significant negative association of the diets net acid load with those variables (3). Higher long-term diet-dependent net acid loads were thus confirmed as a catabolic factor for bone health, although this catabolic effect was apparently overridden by the relatively stronger anabolic effect of protein (3). These findings inspired the hypothesis that the anabolic potential of protein on bone may be further increased by strategies that reduce net acid load (316). This conclusion was supported by the results of a placebo-controlled trial of three hundred and forty-two healthy, elderly men and women over a three-year period. These results showed a supplement of calcium salts of metabolizable organic acids, including citrate, caused a significant increase in total body and femoral neck bone mineral density only in subjects with the highest tertile of protein intake. Conversely, the high protein intake had a positive effect on BMD if (and only if) combined with the supplement (91). Unfortunately, the design of the study does not allow one to distinguish if the positive effect of the supplement was mediated by the increase in calcium supply and/or the reduction in protein-derived acid load by the metabolizable organic acids. The anabolic effect of dietary protein and catabolic effect of the protein-dependent net acid load may explain the conflicting results obtained in numerous epidemiological studies with regard to the effect of protein diets on bone density (reviewed in

184, 316, 293, 264).

Epidemiological studies on the effects of fruits and vegetables

A four-year study of elderly men and women demonstrated that a higher intake of potassium salts of metabolizable organic acids (mostly in the form of fruit and vegetables) was positively correlated with the change in mineral density (359). In several studies on perimenopausal and postmenopausal women, the dietary intake of potassium salts of organic acids was positively correlated with greater bone mineral density, decreased markers of bone resorption, and lower incidence of hip fractures (228, 227, 126, 321). In a study of forty-six subjects with osteopenia or osteoporosis and twenty healthy age- and sex-matched controlled subjects, it was finally shown that a significant proportion of the patients with osteopenia or osteoporosis were associated with incomplete renal tubular acidosis type I (371).

Skeletal muscle wasting as a consequence of low-grade metabolic acidosis

Independent studies from several laboratories have finally shown that metabolic acidosis induces nitrogen wasting associated with increased skeletal muscle protein degradation and loss of lean body mass (240, 252, 125, 239, reviewed in 256). An increased rate of muscle protein degradation under conditions of acidosis has been demonstrated in experimental animals and patients with kidney disease (240, 252) and may be mediated by a glucocorticoid-dependent mechanism (240). The notion that a substantial rate of nitrogen wasting is mediated by the diet-induced, low-grade metabolic acidosis is supported by the finding that supplements of potassium bicarbonate induced a sustained reduction in urinary nitrogen in postmenopausal women (125). A study on nine young, nonsmoking healthy men and women showed that treatment with a combination of potassium carbonate and sodium carbonate caused a decrease in daily urinary excretion of tetrahydrocortisone and significant decrease in plasma cortisol concentration, an important catabolic hormone compromising muscle tissue, in the early morning (239).

Safety (segments of the population that must receive special consideration)

Persons with a heart condition or abnormally low tolerance for dietary potassium should consult their physician. Patients with hyperkalemia or conditions predisposing them to hyperkalemia should not use potassium citrate. It is contraindicated for patients with renal insufficiency. As the excessive rise in urinary pH may promote bacterial growth, urinary pH may be regularly monitored by using pH paper. High doses of alkaline citrates may be avoided. As tripotassium citrate dissolves in water at an alkaline pH, it is recommended to use potassium citrate in a mixture with an amount of citric acid that allows the mixture to dissolve at a neutral pH. This strategy is expected to minimize gastrointestinal complaints that may arise from the alkalinity. It is also recommended to ideally dissolve the daily requirement of alkaline citrates in the daily volume of water or other beverages to avoid drinks with high potassium concentrations (figure 6).

Controversies concerning the effects of alkali salts on the risk of osteoporosis

Several authors from different institutions raised objections against the administration of potassium bicarbonate as a means to prevent or treat menopausal osteoporosis (380, 291, 153). By analogy, these objections would also apply to the use of potassium salts of metabolizable organic acids, including citrate. These concerns should be addressed here. One author raised the question if the observed effect of long-term potassium bicarbonate administration on net acid production, calcium excretion, and bone turnover in postmenopausal women may be relevant to the vast majority of women (380). Specifically, it was argued that the protein content of the women's daily dietary protein (ninety-six grams per sixty kilograms of body weight) in the study in question (318) was considerably higher than that consumed by most women (fifty-five grams per day). However, the authors (317) pointed out that, of the ninety-six gram protein intake per sixty kilograms of body weight, 62 percent was animal, and 38 percent was vegetable protein. They also presented data showing the benefits of potassium bicarbonate were demonstrable also in subjects taking much lower quantities of protein (318). To be on the safe side, potassium citrate and calcium citrate may be used preferentially in combination with high protein diets (0.8 to 1.0 grams per kilogram of body weight per day) or protein supplements. This strategy would take into account the beneficial effects of high protein intake on bone health and intestinal calcium absorption and the important role of the dietary protein intake in the maintenance of muscle mass and muscle function.

Heaney and colleagues (291, 153) reported a study on women showing that subjects with high potassium intakes not only had a reduced urinary calcium excretion but also reduced intestinal calcium absorption, the two effects being of approximately equal magnitude. "Effectively what was gained at the kidney was lost at the gut" (291,153). In the author's response (319), Sebastian and colleagues pointed out that the subjects in the study in question (291) derived their potassium intake mainly from milk and meat rather than fruits and vegetables. These food sources do not contain sufficient amounts of bicarbonate-generating organic acids (319). In any case, all the objections and concerns would be eliminated by combining potassium bicarbonate or, in our case, potassium citrate with an increased protein intake to counter the reduction in intestinal calcium absorption.

Dietary proteins and physical exercise to maintain skeletal muscle mass and function

To maintain an approximately constant protein mass over time, the autophagic protein catabolism during nighttime has to be balanced, on average, by a corresponding amount of protein synthesis during daytime. As skeletal muscle tissues contain approximately 50 percent of all proteins in the human body, they account for most of the autophagic proteolysis and amino acid homeostasis during starvation (213, 374, 238). Old age is typically associated with an involuntary loss of muscle mass (sarcopenia) and muscle function (46, 113, 349), implying the balance between muscular protein catabolism and protein synthesis is less than perfect. After reaching a peak in the third decade of life, skeletal muscle mass is typically lost at a rate of 3 to 8 percent per decade and at an even higher rate after the age of sixty (reviewed in 101). The loss of muscle protein mass in old age is accompanied by a decrease in other proteins, such as plasma albumin (79, 325, 27, 260). Sarcopenia and functional impairment may already start in the fourth decade of life, and substantial sarcopenia is estimated to occur in up to 30 percent of individuals over the age of sixty years (96). Voluntary strength is estimated to decrease by 30 percent between fifty and seventy years of age (203). The loss of muscle mass in old age severely compromises the functional capacity in the elderly, increases the risk of disability, falls, and fractures, and contributes decisively to the loss of quality of life in old age (96). Loss of function affects approximately 7 percent of the elderly over seventy years and approximately 20 percent over eighty years (63, 246). It is estimated that 14 percent of persons between the ages of sixty-five to seventy-five years require assistance with activities of daily living. This figure increases to 45 percent for persons over eighty-five years of age (reviewed in 101). The estimated annual cost of sarcopenia-related health issues to the U.S health care system is more than $18 billion annually (170).

Muscle deterioration resembling human sarcopenia is seen in aging worms (*C. elegans*) and flies (reviewed in 364). The mechanism of sarcopenia is poorly understood, and there is presently no cure. However, there is substantial information about the factors that regulate muscular protein synthesis and certain strategies that improve the balance between protein breakdown and protein synthesis. The principle requirement for protein synthesis is the adequate supply of biosynthetic precursor amino acids that are normally derived from dietary proteins. An inadequate dietary intake of protein frequently contributes to the development of sarcopenia (17, 66, 224). Even in Western countries, protein-energy malnutrition is commonly seen in the elderly (4). Based on nitrogen balance studies, the RDA for both men and women is currently 0.8 grams of good quality protein per kilogram of body weight per day (271). A recommendation based on studies of skeletal muscle metabolism and function would probably have been more meaningful (378). Several authors agree that the elderly should consume more protein than 0.8 grams of good quality protein per kilogram of body weight per day. Healthy, elderly men and women between fifty-five and seventy-seven years of age showed a decrease in mid-thigh muscle area and decrease in urinary nitrogen excretion consistent with metabolic accommodation when provided with this amount of protein during a fourteen-week precisely controlled diet study (60). One study showed that resistance exercise results in a decrease in nitrogen excretion (114), suggesting either an adaptation to inadequate protein availability or greater efficiency in protein utilization during such exercise programs. There is no evidence that a mere increase in protein intake may be sufficient to prevent the problem of aging-related sarcopenia. The available evidence suggests an increase in dietary protein intake can only prevent the consequences of malnutrition, not the age-related loss in muscle protein. Under certain conditions, dietary protein supplementation may be effective in slowing or even reversing the loss in muscle mass and muscle function. This book is not intended to serve as a complete and unbiased review of the field. But it provides the basic information and arguments that support a specific recommendation.

Regulation of protein synthesis at the molecular level

Muscular protein synthesis is regulated at the translational level by the availability of free amino acids (reviewed in 187, 195). The integrating point for the insulin receptor signaling cascade and action of amino acids is the mammalian target of rapamycin (mTOR), which is also critically involved in the negative regulation of autophagy (figure 3). mTOR is upregulated by increasing concentrations of leucine and a small group of other amino acids collectively called regulatory amino acids (257).

Effect of dietary protein and amino acid administration on protein synthesis in vivo

In line with these molecular mechanisms, it was found that amino acid infusion in the fasted state rapidly increases muscle protein synthesis in humans, even in the absence of prior exercise (365). Several studies have shown that feeding of mixed amino acids or protein in combination with the free amino acid leucine and carbohydrate increases muscle protein synthesis in both young and elderly subjects (365, 366, 295, 276, 367, 194). Feeding branched-chain amino acids was shown to increase both global and specific mRNA translation (188). The leucine- and cysteine-rich whey protein was shown to stimulate protein synthesis in young and elderly subjects and proved to be more effective than casein (89, 90). The difference between the effects of whey protein and casein was even stronger in seventy-two-year-olds than in twenty-four-year-old volunteers (90). Another study on young healthy volunteers also showed that whey protein was more effective than casein in stimulating muscle net protein synthesis (353).

The fast digestion rate of the whey protein might have been at least partially responsible for the observed difference because pulse feeding caused a more positive nitrogen balance than a spread pattern in which the same intake was evenly distributed over four meals (12). Ingestion of a single meal of whey protein by healthy adults induces a strong, but brief, increase in plasma amino acids, whereas a single casein meal induces a prolonged, but only moderately elevated, plateau of amino acids (figure 18) (37, 88, 90). Notably, the high peak concentrations of leucine may be important for the stimulation of protein synthesis in the elderly as these are less responsive to lower leucine concentrations than young adults (90, 180). But the high peak amino acid concentrations after the whey protein meal come at the price that a greater proportion of the amino acids were metabolized in pathways other than protein synthesis if compared with the casein meal (38, 88). Physical exercise immediately before or after the whey protein meal can be expected to ameliorate this effect by increasing the clearance rate of amino acids from the blood into the muscle tissues. In a study on the stimulation of mTOR and S6K1 after endurance exercise in rats, whey protein was also more effective than soy protein (10), which is another fast protein (40) but known to contain less leucine.

In line with the stimulation of protein synthesis, one study in healthy, young subjects confined to bed rest showed that the increased availability of amino acids increases both muscle mass and strength, even in the complete absence of muscular activity (275).

Potential adverse effects of a high dietary protein intake

Little is known about adverse effects of excessive protein intakes. While an upper limit for total protein in the diet was set at no more than 30 percent of total energy intake, there were insufficient data to provide dose-response relationships to establish a Tolerable Upper Intake Level (UL) for total protein or any of the amino acids (271). One of the trivial negative consequences of high protein consumption is the fat intake that results from the high fat content of the most common dietary protein sources. This problem can be balanced by focusing on fat-free foods. Another adverse effect, the generation of metabolic acids by sulfur-containing proteins, can be ameliorated by carefully balancing the protein intake with the dietary intake of alkali compounds, as described previously. A more subtle consequence of high protein intakes is the induction of insulin resistance in humans by high physiological levels of amino acids (197, 357).

A less well-investigated point of major concern is that the stimulatory effect of protein consumption on the endogenous protein synthesis may cause an undesirable hypertrophy of tissues other than skeletal muscle. Studies in different experimental animal species indicated that high dietary protein levels caused a weight gain of the kidney, thymus, and, to a lesser extent, liver (223, 182, 67, 183, 122). Clinical studies have shown that a portion of ingested amino acids is not available to the muscle tissue due to the splanchnic bed utilization (mainly protein synthesis and amino acid breakdown and oxidation in the liver; figure 15). This portion increases with age, indicating older adults take up more amino acids by the liver than young individuals (38, 385). As vascular smooth muscle cell proliferation and hyperplasia has been implicated in aging-related vascular diseases (268, 55), there is the alarming possibility that high-protein diets may account for some of the age-related changes in the vascular smooth muscle cells of the arteries and lead to arterial stiffening and thickening. The increase in prostate volume in elderly men is another example of an undesirable hypertrophy of a muscle tissue. Although the effects of dietary protein intakes on various undesirable forms of tissue hypertrophy are generally not well-investigated, it is desirable to target the stimulatory effects of dietary protein intake, preferentially, to the protein synthesis in skeletal muscle tissues. Physical exercise appears to be the best method to serve this purpose. Together with protein supplementation, it is also the most effective way to increase skeletal muscle mass and muscle function in old age.

Effects of physical exercise on muscle protein synthesis, muscle mass, and muscle function

Several studies have shown that resistance-type exercise can effectively stimulate muscle protein synthesis (70, 230, 229, 285, 35, 376, 381). Both resistance and endurance exercises were shown to stimulate protein synthesis at the level of translation initiation in synergy with low (fasting) levels of insulin (reviewed in 187). More recently, a six-month resistance exercise training program was shown to significantly change the expression of certain genes associated with mitochondrial function, which were most strongly affected by age (245).

Physical exercise is also the best-investigated and scientifically proven method to increase both skeletal muscle function and muscle mass. Notably, resistance exercise can increase muscle mass and muscle function in older adults, even into the ninth decade of life (117). Resistance exercise training in elderly and very old adults was shown to induce significant increases in muscle mass (8), muscle size (117, 130), muscle strength (62), and mitochondrial function (245). An even more effective exercise for functional task performance in old age may be the recently developed high-velocity power training that trains specifically muscle power, that is, the ability to produce force quickly (reviewed in 311). The American College of Medicine recommended a well-rounded training program, including aerobic and resistance training together with flexibility exercises, for maintaining muscular strength and endurance and flexibility of the major muscle groups (287). Disuse is one of the factors that have been implicated in the process of muscle loss, whereas long-term physical activity is associated with a reduction in morbidity and mortality in humans (277).

Effect of protein intake together with exercise on muscle protein synthesis and function

The stimulation of protein synthesis by exercise can be amplified by amino acids or protein (33, 353). Notably, intravenous infusion of amino acids postexercise (33) or consumption of proteins or amino acid supplements immediately before or immediately after resistance exercise was shown to strongly enhance the anabolic response to the exercise activity by increasing protein synthesis and net protein balance compared to control treatments (350, 351, 39, 249, 294, 352, 353). Maximum skeletal muscle hypertrophy and increase in isokinetic strength were found when protein was supplemented immediately after exercise, but not two hours after exercise (111).

Despite the significant effects of protein or amino acid feeding on protein synthesis, attempts to enhance the effects of resistance training on muscle functions by protein or amino acid supplementation yielded mixed and, essentially, sobering results (59, 118, 375, 5, 9). Dietary supplementation of branched-chain amino acids improved endurance and muscle power in young canoeists (83), but failed to augment the anabolic response to exercise training in another study (129). Several studies involving various types of proteins in combination with resistance exercise programs over a period of ten to fifty weeks generally showed the protein supplements had little or no effect on skeletal muscle strength, even though it caused a significant increase in muscle size in some of the studies (118, 247, 8, 61, 301, 661, 47, 5).

This series of rather sobering results has lead to the conclusion that protein-enriched nutritional supplements do not influence training-induced improvements when adequate dietary protein above the RDA of 0.8 grams per kilogram of body weight per day is consumed (58, 195).

However, impressive synergistic effects between protein supplementation and exercise programs have been obtained in certain special conditions. In a study on elderly men between seventy and eighty years of age, it was found that supplementation with a mix of skim milk-derived and soy bean proteins, in combination with carbohydrate and lipids, caused an increase in isokinetic strength and mean fiber area only if applied immediately but not two hours after each training session (111). Two studies on healthy, young subjects revealed that high doses of whey protein, in combination with resistance training over a period of ten and six weeks, respectively, yielded a significantly greater improvement in strength than either casein or placebo, respectively (82, 48). In both studies, the volunteers consumed four doses of supplement distributed over the day, corresponding to a total amount of one hundred grams per eighty kilograms of body weight or ninety-six grams per eighty kilograms of body weight, respectively. Similarly, undenatured whey protein (Immunocal) significantly increased peak power and "30 s work capacity" in a whole-leg isokinetic cycle test if compared with placebo-treated control subjects in a randomized, double-blind study of young, healthy subjects (202).

In another study on young, healthy subjects, it was found the dose of thirty-two grams of whey protein per eighty kilograms of body weight over a ten-week period mediated a significantly greater increase in lean body mass and strength if given immediately before and after the exercise period, as compared to the same dose given in the morning and late evening (81).

--

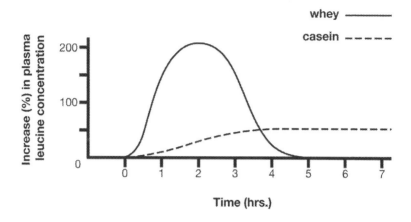

Fig. 17. Increase in plasma amino acid (leucine) concentration after ingestion of whey protein or casein (schematic illustration). Relative increase (%) in plasma leucine concentrations after a single meal of whey protein or casein (schematic illustration of findings from references 36, 87, and 89).

Taken together, these studies suggest that, for slowing the rate of aging, whey protein may possibly be a most useful dietary protein for three different reasons.

1. The brief, but high, temporary increase in plasma amino acid concentrations after a single meal of whey protein (figure 17), in combination with its relatively high leucine content, makes this protein ideally suited to increase muscle protein synthesis, muscle mass, and muscle function. As intense physical exercise induces a particularly strong demand for amino acids in the period around and immediately after exercise, it is most reasonable to consume the whey protein immediately before and/or after exercise so the brief peak of high amino acid concentrations coincides with the maximum amino acid demand of the skeletal muscle tissues. Using this protocol, the stimulatory effects of the high leucine concentration on protein synthesis seems to synergize best with the stimulatory effect of exercise.

2. By consuming whey protein immediately before and/or after physical exercise, a relatively high proportion of its amino acids

is being used for skeletal muscle protein synthesis instead of stimulating undesirable hypertrophy in other tissues. A strong enhancement of the anabolic effect of exercise was also found if very high doses of whey proteins were given at four different time points during the day. But, in this case, the doses taken at time points distant to the exercise period were presumably irrelevant for the exercise-induced anabolic effect and likely to favor undesirable protein synthesis in hypertrophic tissues other than skeletal muscle because whey protein taken in the early morning or late evening (times distant to the exercise period) did not enhance the anabolic effect of exercise.

3. The use of the cysteine-rich whey protein at doses between ten and thirty grams per day (equivalent to approximately 0.27 to 0.8 grams of cysteine) as a regular component of the dietary protein would have the additional advantage that it provides the extra amount of cysteine that can be expected to ameliorate the vicious cycle of oxidative stress illustrated in figure 5. The failure of frail, elderly patients with low postabsorptive plasma cysteine and asparagine concentrations to benefit from physical exercise, unless supplemented with an additional source of cysteine, suggests the elderly benefit from both components of the whey protein, the high cysteine and leucine content. A moderate amount of slow proteins may, nonetheless, be useful to minimize muscle protein breakdown during daytime (33, 37, 90). A moderate amount of whey protein in the morning may help to replenish the low cysteine and glutathione pools after overnight starvation.

The available evidence suggests that elderly with a sedentary life style may have an unfavorable ratio of skeletal muscle protein synthesis versus undesirable protein synthesis in vascular smooth muscle cells and other tissues. Without physical exercise these persons may have an unfavorable prognosis regardless whether they consume protein or whether they starve and derive their amino acids from skeletal muscle atrophy.

Chapter Eight

General Conclusions

The Paradigm

Self-rejuvenation works best if periods of autophagy, that is self-cannibalism, alternate with periods of reconstruction to refill the gaps. Ideally, one may want to use every minute of ones life to support either one or the other in the most rigorous way. However, whereas most people intuitively place more emphasis on the constructive aspect (for example on body building), the combined evidence from numerous studies on longevity consistently shows that "self-cannibalism" and related functions are the more critical requirements for a long life span. These important processes happen mainly during periods of starvation. In humans they happen at night.

Taken together, there are strong reasons to believe the normal life span of man and most animals is limited primarily by an oxidative spiral (figure 5/figure 10) that can be viewed as the first cause of death. This vicious cycle includes a decrease in the intracellular glutathione level, various manifestations of oxidative stress, aberrant activation of the insulin signaling mechanism during periods of starvation, and decline in autophagic activity. As a controlled mechanism of self-destruction, autophagy is critically involved in the removal and recycling of cellular waste, which is required for the rejuvenation of cellular structures and maintenance of adequate free amino acid levels under starving conditions. Both of these functions deteriorate in old age. One of the well-documented consequences in man is the age-related decline of the plasma cysteine concentration under starving conditions, which leads to a decrease in glutathione levels. This facilitates the development of oxidative stress and accumulation of oxidative damage.

The cycle in figure 5 provides a unifying explanation for two seemingly very different sets of longevity mutants, that is, one group of mutants with a defect in the insulin signaling mechanism and another group that expresses an increased capacity to scavenge oxygen radicals and/or hydrogen peroxide. This vicious cycle is inevitably integrated in a larger physiological network in the sense it can affect numerous other biological processes and may itself be affected by other processes. The substantial life span extension in two groups of markedly different longevity strains of animals suggests the autonomous progression of this cycle is the primary cause of death in a broad range of animal species.

Taken together, these findings have led to a combination of practical interventions designed to strengthen the autophagic activity in old age. Although these interventions involve components of our regular diet, these substances have quasi-pharmacological activities and should be used in a well-balanced way. Whenever possible, diagnostic tools have been described to provide guidelines for these interventions. Rapamycin is a drug that was recently shown to prolong the life span of mice which started receiving this treatment at an age corresponding to 60 years in humans. As rapamycin inhibits TOR/mTOR, a key element in the oxidative cycle (figure 10), it inevitably inhibits TOR/mTOR-dependent synthetic processes after food intake (figure 3).

Any program that strengthens the autophagic activity should be combined with a complementary program that strengthens the synthetic activities and compensates for the losses caused by the autophagic protein catabolism. Whatever lifestyle one may look at there is arguably no person in the world who optimally uses the circadian cycle of the day to sequentially maximize both the autophagic activity and the synthetic activity which only in combination ensure structural turnover and rejuvenation. This book may help to improve both types of activities.

Current Opinions of Other Authors in Aging Research

What is novel about these assessments and recommendations? In general, these assessments are in agreement with current opinions in aging research and recent reviews including the excellent review by Vijg and Campisi (364). In view of the substantial life span extension in various longevity strains of worms, flies, and mice, there is a general consensus about the importance of insulin signaling and IGF-1 signaling activities, the FOXO transcription factors, and role of ROS in aging. After decades of skepticism, there is now a cautious tendency to admit there is no scientific reason for not striving to cure aging. Extending the human life span by a finite margin may be even a more realistic goal than curing all aspects of aging.

Some important aspects, however, have not previously been taken into consideration. Because of the dominance of genetic methods in aging-research, such as the use of mutants and knockout animals, spatiotemporal aspects have been largely dismissed. The fact that certain gene products, such as the components of the insulin signaling pathway, may have different roles at different time points has been largely ignored. Also, in the recent study on the effects of rapamycin in mice by Harrison et al. (chapter 5) this drug was added to the food, that means it was delivered in the postprandial state. Vijg and Campisi (364) deserve to be credited for acknowledging this problem, at least in principle, when they discuss the differential roles of IGF-1 signaling during early adulthood versus old age. But the differential roles of the insulin signaling pathway during the circadian cycle have still been underappreciated. According to the wealth of information summarized here, the differential physiological conditions during daytime and nighttime (that is, the circadian cycle) play an absolutely crucial role in the aging process.

Finally, most reviews on aging have given virtually no consideration to the aging-related change in amino acid homeostasis and its relevance to cellular levels of glutathione, that is, the quantitatively most important antioxidant in cells and tissues. Discussions about antioxidants have been mainly limited to vitamins C and E, ß-carotene, resveratrol and synthetic ROS scavengers (364). This reflects the fact that aging-related changes in endogenous antioxidant and metabolite levels are currently less appreciated by the scientific community than structural changes in genes, proteins, or other cellular constituents. This book, in contrast emphasizes the possibility that aging may be largely determined by a change in metabolite levels, that is, a change in software rather than hardware. This possibility (and notably the inherent aspect of reversibility) provides an opportunity that should not be dismissed. Changes in metabolite concentrations may even be used as biomarkers to characterize the degenerative process of aging.

The interventions proposed in this book are not meant to substitute for the current recommendations toward a healthy and physically active lifestyle. One is still advised to watch one's weight, eat adequate amounts of vitamins, fruits, vegetables, omega-3 fatty acids, and so forth. *Dietary Reference Intakes* by the Institute of Medicine of the National Academies, *Prescription for Nutritional Healing* by Phyllis Balch (2006), *The Role of Protein and Amino Acids in Sustaining and Enhancing Performance* (77), or other similar publications are still useful reading. But it is time to look beyond these recommendations and give more attention to the emerging mechanisms of aging and conclusions described in this book.

Critical Assessment of the Evidence and Choices

Key to the concept of the cycle in figure 5 was the finding that the age-related decline in glutathione concentrations is associated with an age-related decline of its precursor amino acid cysteine and simultaneous decline of the seemingly unrelated amino acid asparagine. The decrease in both cysteine and asparagine indicate a change in amino acid homeostasis, a function that is controlled by the autophagic protein catabolism and possibly other forms of insulin sensitive mechanisms of protein catabolism. In view of the relatively low plasma concentrations of cysteine and its relatively higher representation in muscle proteins, a relatively small shift in autophagic activity is to be expected to yield a relatively strong decrease in postabsorptive plasma cysteine and intracellular glutathione concentrations. The decline in the postabsorptive plasma concentrations of both cysteine and asparagine can potentially serve as a diagnostic tool (biomarker) to assess the level of postabsorptive autophagic activity and indirectly the state of the cycle in a given individual. The decrease in reduced cysteine as a critical precursor of glutathione biosynthesis is clearly the biologically more relevant parameter but technically more difficult to measure than asparagine.

Some of the key studies cited in support of this concept need to be repeated. In addition there are gaps of information, notably in the section on protein intake. But one simply has the choice to either take action on the basis of the present state of knowledge or wait for more and better evidence to come.

Summary of the Recommended Interventions

Calorie restriction is an intervention that should be considered in the context of this program because it was shown to increase autophagic activity and life span in animal studies. However, as massive calorie restriction may not be appealing to most, it is suggested to restrict the intake of calories only to the point where the skeletal muscle mass and muscle function is not compromised. Persons who are regularly performing physical exercise would be the first to notice negative changes in their performance.

Cysteine supplementation is recommended to ameliorate the age-related oxidative stress. In view of the vicious cycle of figure 5, one may want to increase the dietary cysteine intake to the point where the original level of autophagic activity is reestablished and an adequate (youthful) postabsorptive plasma cysteine level can be maintained by autophagic breakdown of endogenous protein sources. Unfortunately, this may be difficult to achieve (see chapter 5). Also, there are no simple diagnostic tests to monitor the rate of autophagic activity. In the absence of a better test, the postabsorptive cysteine and asparagine levels may serve as the least invasive measurements to monitor the individual state of the vicious cycle. Occasional measurements of the postabsorptive glucose levels may also serve as a crude guideline that gives some information about changes in the postabsorptive insulin receptor signaling activity. More detailed guidelines are given in the addendum.

The cysteine-rich whey protein appears to be ideally suited for cysteine supplementation because it can serve two purposes at the same time. At a daily dose of ten to thirty grams consumed immediately after some form of physical exercise, dietary whey protein can be expected to substantially improve muscle protein synthesis and muscle function and simultaneously meet the increased demand for cysteine to ameliorate the age-related oxidative stress.

To further increase the availability of free cysteine in the plasma and muscle tissue during the early morning hours, it is recommended to combine the dietary cysteine supplementation with the method of *water-assisted autophagy*, a simple and mild intervention designed to increase the autophagic protein catabolism and release of free cysteine notably in the late night and early morning hours. One can expect to achieve this effect simply by drinking one hundred to five hundred milliliters of water during the night approximately two to three hours before breakfast. A disadvantage of this method is the need to wake up in the middle of the night. But, in the absence of better and well-established methods to enhance autophagy, this method, in combination with cysteine supplementation, may be the best (and notably nonpharmacological) method available.

The dietary carbohydrate intake should be moderate and evenly distributed over the day. One of the important quasi-pharmacological effects of our dietary carbohydrate intake is to avoid the undesirable condition of hypoglycemia. It may be most reasonable to essentially follow the same recommendation that is typically given to diabetic patients, that is, to distribute the daily dietary carbohydrate consumption evenly throughout the day by consuming small amounts of carbohydrate approximately every two hours (figure 13). Any excess dietary carbohydrate intake is a risk factor for the development of obesity and diabetes. By triggering the production of insulin, the daily dietary carbohydrate intake typically limits the time window during which autophagy can proceed.

The dietary intake of creatine should also be moderate. As creatine supplementation was shown to reverse the inhibitory effect of cysteine supplementation on the basic (postabsorptive) insulin signaling activity, creatine consumption should be well-balanced. A regular high dietary intake of meat, meat extracts, chicken soup, or creatine supplements should be avoided. A consistently low dietary creatine intake may also be avoided because it is incompatible with maximum muscle size and muscle force. A more specific recommendation is described in addendum one.

As magnesium ATP is a key substrate for the insulin receptor kinase a reduced magnesium availability compromises the insulin receptor signaling cascade. However, as magnesium is critically involved in many physiological processes, it is not recommended to use magnesium restriction as a tool to derepress autophagic activity. The RDA of magnesium is four hundred and twenty milligrams per day for men and three hundred and twenty milligrams per day for women. Magnesium supplementation may be particularly important in periods of calorie restriction.

Persons with diets high in cysteine-rich proteins or other forms of cysteine supplementation need to compensate for the resulting acid load. In view of the increase in metabolic acid production and its potential effect on BMD and osteoporosis, it is reasonable to combine an increased consumption of dietary cysteine-rich proteins with an adequate dietary supplement that compensates for the acid load. An increase in the consumption of fruit and vegetables would reduce the degree of acidification and improve the general health condition, but the necessary major changes in dietary habits are not likely to occur soon. Increasing the consumption of fruit and vegetables also means increasing the consumption of carbohydrates. Dietary supplementation of potassium and calcium citrates may be the best alternative. These citric acid salts may be dissolved in tea, fruit juices, or water and distributed over the day (figure 13). Postmenopausal women are obviously the group that would benefit most from the use of alkaline or earth alkali citrates. However, as bone loss begins already between the ages of eighteen and thirty years and as osteoporosis is also observed (although less commonly) in men, it is recommended that all persons with a urine pH less than or equal to 6.5 may benefit from such supplements. With appropriate pH paper slips, even an untrained person can easily determine his or her urine pH and adjust the dose of supplement in such a way that the urine pH is increased to a value between approximately 6.5 and 6.8. No additional benefit is expected if the urine pH exceeds the value of 6.8. The dietary supplement is not recommended for persons with a urine pH greater than or equal to 6.8. Persons with a heart condition may consult their doctor before using potassium citrate.

The recommendation for the dietary protein consumption is primarily designed to compensate for the autophagic loss of protein mass by a corresponding amount of protein synthesis. In view of the normal age-related loss of muscle protein and muscle function, this is the most difficult part of the program.

The cysteine- and leucine-rich whey protein was found to be more effective than casein or soy protein and is therefore the ideal dietary protein source to support the maintenance of skeletal muscle mass and muscle function, especially in old age. To shift nutrient utilization in favor of skeletal muscle tissues and against undesirable forms of tissue hypertrophy, whey protein should ideally be consumed immediately before and/or after physical exercise. In this case, the short time window of maximum exercise-induced skeletal muscle protein synthesis coincides well with the maximum availability of the amino acids in the plasma, which reaches a temporary and relatively high peak already two hours after whey protein consumption. Ideally, a person of eighty kilograms of body weight should consume about ten to thirty grams of whey protein immediately before or after exercise. This is incidentally an adequate amount of cysteine supplementation to ameliorate the vicious cycle of figure 5. An additional small amount of the cysteine-rich whey protein may be consumed in the morning to account for the relatively low plasma cysteine and intracellular glutathione levels in the starved state (figure 13). The rest of the daily protein intake may be distributed over the day. The total protein consumption per day should be slightly higher than the RDA of 0.8 grams per kilogram of body weight, but may be slightly lower on days with little physical activity. Admittedly, this schedule of protein intake is inconvenient as it is incompatible with the eating habits in most Western countries. Food intake is typically a social event and organized during traditional hours of the day.

Scientific evidence underscores the importance of physical exercise. If someone in the seventh decade of life considers it painful or simply uninteresting to spend time in the fitness club or if he or she decides to quit the longtime favorite sport simply for lack of enthusiasm, he or she should know this is not only a question of lifting the heavy suitcase more or less easily. It is a question of how to age, and it determines the quality of life in the years to come. By voluntarily decreasing the exercise intensity, one enters a vicious cycle that eventually leads to a decrease in exercise capacity and further involuntary decrease in exercise intensity (figure 18). The amount of protein intake should be adjusted to the individual body weight and the amount of exercise.

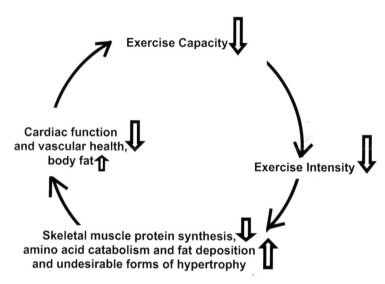

Fig. 18. Vicious cycle compromising skeletal muscle protein synthesis and favoring undesirable forms of hypertrophy. A voluntary or involuntary decrease in exercise intensity leads to a decrease in skeletal muscle protein synthesis and a correspondingly increased conversion of amino acids into body fat and undesirable protein synthesis in other cells and tissues. Such undesirable forms of hypertrophy may contribute to the age-related change in heart weight, vascular health, and body fat, which then compromises the exercise capacity and intensity.

Critical Assessment of Key Recommendations

Moderately restricting the caloric intake is basically in line with the general recommendation to watch one's weight. This is supported by general experience. Addendum one describes specific recommendations for a more pronounced calorie restriction. By describing some of the mechanisms by which calorie restriction acts upon the mechanism of aging and specifically on the vicious cycle of figure 5, it is hoped these pages will help to raise the general acceptance and compliance. Essentially, the same applies to the recommendations:

- Distribute the carbohydrate consumption evenly over the day in relatively small amounts and small time intervals
- Avoid an excessive use of creatine and restrict the consumption of creatine-containing foods such as beef
- Engage in regular physical exercise

The recommendation to use supplements of potassium citrate is based upon the belief that the most reasonable and widely known recommendation to eat enough fruit and vegetables will never meet with sufficient compliance. The consumption of citric acid salts may be a more acceptable alternative to achieve an adequate acid-base balance.

Water-assisted autophagy as a recommendation to enhance the autophagic activity during the night is a novel but unproven method that targets mTOR, the same regulatory element which is targeted by rapamycin. Because the consumption of clean water is generally considered as safe, one may simply try this method with gradually increasing volumes and determine the perceived benefits.

Cysteine supplementation is another tool designed to suppress the oxidative spiral of figure 5/figure 10 and slow the increase in oxidative stress and aging-related degenerative processes. This method is based on a substantial amount of clinical and laboratory evidence, but still largely unknown to the general public. It deserves a wider public awareness. Cysteine supplementation by consumption of cysteine-rich whey proteins has the additional advantage that these proteins, if used optimally in conjunction with physical exercise, may provide the best means to slow the loss of muscle function in old age.

The Practical Message

If seen with a birds-eye-view, self-rejuvenation involves alternating periods of regulated self-destruction as a means of waste removal and periods of reconstruction to compensate for the losses. Taken together it is suggested that the quality of life in old age and the maximum human life span may be increased by a set of interventions designed to maximize the autophagic activity during the night while strengthening synthetic activities during the day. As even with the best interventions autophagic and synthetic activities per time unit are limited, it may require a carefully designed protocol throughout the circadian cicle of the day to achieve optimal results. Nobody can be expected to comply perfectly to such an uncomfortable procedure. To strictly follow all recommendations outlined in the previous sections, one would have to show the level of dedication and discipline of a top athlete. *The rate of aging is therefore largely determined by the brain.* However, in contrast to the rigorous programs of calorie restriction that some voluntarily practice, the recommendations given here do not involve a major sacrifice. If the reader becomes familiar with the underlying mechanisms and benefits, he or she may find the incentive to comply at least to some extent. Even the non-scientist may benefit from glancing through the scientific evidence sections.

It may be surprising to see the recommended interventions involve not more than a thoughtful if inconvenient way of using our daily foodstuff. Can such a seemingly trivial set of interventions really do much of a difference? It may be worthwhile to look at the following example. If an untrained person is given a golf club and ball, he or she will find it difficult to hit the ball as far as one hundred yards whereas the professional will easily reach three hundred yards or more. It needs only the detailed knowledge of the mechanisms that allows the expert to get the extra distance. This may also apply to the use of foodstuff. Based on the life span extension in various animals, there is good reason to believe that one can achieve a substantial extra distance in terms of longevity and quality of life in old age simply by applying better strategies in using daily foodstuff.

As all of these recommendations involve components of the normal human foodstuff in combination with adequate physical activity, one may wonder if one or the other person in the past may have used all these components either intuitively or simply by chance. Can one really expect to *increase* the *maximum* human life span? The answer is that probably nobody has ever observed the rigorous procedures described above, and some of the ingredients such as citric acid salts, purified whey proteins, or other enriched sources of cysteine were simply not available until recently. There is a good chance that man can now advance to a higher level of longevity and quality of life in old age.

This set of recommendations has to be seen only as a start of an open-ended initiative. More science-based recommendations designed to slow the vicious cycle of figure 5 are likely to follow. The use of low doses of rapamycin before sleeping may soon become common practice, once clinical data on safety will become available. Moreover, with a more detailed understanding of the underlying mechanisms one may reasonably expect to see in the very near future markedly more effective strategies given the fact that all the life extending strategies identified so far , including calorie restriction, mutations in the insulin signaling pathway or the addition of rapamycin to the food, have substantial adverse effects. The development of new interventions will be complemented by the development of additional noninvasive methods to monitor the state of the vicious cycle of figure 5.

A special challenge is, that key processes of self-rejuvenation, notably the autophagic functions of waste removal and amino acid homeostasis and their inhibition by redox-sensitive components of the insulin signaling cascade, are mainly happening in the starved condition during the night and early morning hours. To selectively target this time period in genetic or therapeutic studies is a formidable challenge. Future studies are likely to give more attention to interventions that act upon this time period. The method of water-assisted autophagy is only a first step along this line. The effects of antioxidant vitamins C and E and of cysteine supplementation in previous studies on aging might have been limited by the fact that these supplements have typically been given during the day with little consequence for the cysteine and glutathione availability at night and in the early morning hours. Slow-release formulas may provide a better solution. This may also apply to studies on the effects of rapamycin and related drugs on the rate of aging in mice (see addendum two). There is obviously room for improvement.

Chapter Nine

Future Perspective

Assuming the mutations in the insulin receptor signaling cascade of the longevity mutants eliminated a first cause of death that limits the life span of a wide range of animal species, it would be of practical interest to determine in a second step if certain double mutants can be isolated with an even more extended life span. This kind of strategy may possibly reveal a second cause of death and then possibly a third one and so on. Studies on various aging-related degenerative processes in several laboratories have already indicated that other potential causes of death do exist. For practical purposes, it would be interesting to know their place in a hierarchy of relevance. There is reason to believe that a detailed knowledge of these mechanisms will not only help us to increase the human life span but also (and more importantly) improve the quality of life in old age.

Glossary

- The terms *first cause of death* and *principal cause of death* are (synonymously) defined in this book as the lethal mechanism that limits the maximum human life span. The term "first" is based on the discovery of longevity mutants of animals with markedly extended life span in which one mechanism of death (first cause of death) appears to be inactivated, thereby exposing a somewhat slower *second cause of death*.

- The *maximum human life span* is the life span of the oldest human and is approximately one hundred and twenty years. It is to be distinguished from the average human life span.

- *Amino acids* are small molecules that serve as the brick stones from which proteins are formed.

- *Proteins* are the quantitatively most important building blocks of cells and tissues and carriers of important biological functions. Different proteins contain different sequences of amino acids.

- *Membranes* are continuous sheets consisting mainly of proteins and lipids (fat molecules). Membranes separate different parts of the intracellular space and the inside from the outside.

- *Organelles* are organ-like structures with special biological functions that are found in almost all cells of living organisms. Organelles consist mainly of proteins and lipids. In old age, cells often show a conspicuous accumulation of damaged organelles.

- *Autophagy* (literally self-eating) is a mechanism of controlled self-destruction. It is the main mechanism by which damaged organelles can be removed from cells and tissues and make room for new and functionally intact structures.

- *Regulatory amino acids* such as leucine are involved in downregulating the autophagic activity and upregulating protein synthesis in a concentration-dependent way.

- The *postabsorptive* (fasted) state is a state of starvation that typically occurs in the night and early morning hours in humans. It is characterized by low amino acid levels in the blood. It is the state in which autophagic activity is most strongly expressed.

- *Cysteine* is a sulfur-containing amino acid and the most limiting precursor for the biosynthesis of glutathione.

- *Glutathione* is a molecule consisting of cysteine and two other amino acids, glycine and glutamate. Glutathione is the quantitatively most important scavenger of oxygen radicals and therefore an important defense against radical-mediated oxidative damage.

- *Oxygen radicals* are chemically highly aggressive molecules derived from atmospheric oxygen. They interact with many cellular components and cause structural damage. Oxygen radicals are the most prominent subgroup among the widely known free radicals.

- *Oxidative stress* is a condition mediated by elevated tissue levels of oxygen radicals and related chemically aggressive molecules.

Bibliography

1. Abeliovich, H., and D.J. Klionsky. 2001. Autophagy in yeast: mechanistic insights and physiological functions. *Mol Biol Rev* 65:463–479.

2. Adams, N.D., R.W. Gray, and J. Lemann Jr. 1979. The calciuria of increased fixed acid production in humans: Evidence against a role for parathyroid hormone and 1, 25-(OH)$_2$ –vitamin D. *Calcif Tissue Int* 27:233–239.

3. Alexy, U, T. Remer, F. Manz, C.M. Neu, and E. Schoenau. 2005. Long-term protein intake and dietary potential renal acid load are associated with bone modeling and remodeling at the proximal radius in healthy children. *Am J Clin Nutr* 82:1107–1114.

4. Allison, S.P. 1995. Cost-effectiveness of nutritional support in the elderly. *Proc Nutr Soc* 54:693–699.

5. Andersen, L.L., G. Tufekovic, M.K. Zebis, R.M. Crameri, G. Verlaan, M. Kjaer, C. Suetta, P. Magnusson, and P. Aagaard. 2005. The effect of resistance training combined with timed ingestion of protein on muscle fiber size and muscle strength. *Metabolism* 54:151–156.

6. Anderson, T.J., A. Uehata, and M.D. Gerhard. 1995. Close relation of endothelial function in the human coronary and peripheral circulations. *J Am Coll Cardiol* 26:1235–1241.

7. Andrews, N.P., A. Prasad, and A.A. Quyyumi. 2001.

N-acetylcysteine improves coronary and peripheral vascular function. *J Am Coll Cardiol* 37:117–123.

8. Andrews, R.D., D.A. MacLean, and S.E. Riechman. 2006. Protein intake for skeletal muscle hypertrophy with resistance training in seniors. *Int J Sport Nutr Exerc Metab* 16:362–372.

9. Andziak, B., T.P. O'Connor, W.Qi, E.M. DeWaal, A. Pierce, A.R. Chaudhuri, H. Van Remmen, and R. Buffenstein. 2006. High oxidative damage levels in the longest-living rodent, the naked mole-rat. *Aging Cell* 5:463–471.

10. Anthony, T.G., B.J. McDaniel, P. Knoll, B. Piyawan, G.L. Paul, and M.A. McNurlan. 2007. Feeding meals containing soy or whey protein after exercise stimulates protein synthesis and translation initiation in the skeletal muscle of male rats. *J Nutr* 137:357–362.

11. Arivazhagan, P., K. Ramanathan, and C. Panneerselvam. 2001. Effect of DL-alpha-lipoic acid on mitochondrial enzymes in aged rats. *Chem Biol Interact* 138:189–198.

12. Arnal, M.A., L. Mosoni, Y. Boirie, M.L. Houlier, L. Morin, E. Verdier, P. Ritz, J.M. Antoine, J. Prugnaud, P.P. Beaufrère. 1999. Protein pulse feeding improves protein retention in elderly women. *Am J Clin Nutr* 69:1202–1208.

13. Arnett, T.R., and D.W. Dempster. 1986. Effect of pH on bone resorption by rat osteoclasts *in vitro*. *Endocrinology* 119:119–124.

14. Arosio, E., S. De Marchi, M. Zannoni, M. Prior, and A. Lechi. 2002. Effect of glutathione infusion on leg arterial circulation, cutaneous microcirculation, and pain-free walking distance in patients with peripheral obstructive arterial disease: A randomized, double-blind, placebo-controlled trial. *Mayo Clin Proc* 77:754–759.

15. Ashfaq, S., J.L. Abramson, D.P. Jones, S.D. Rhodes, W.S. Weintraub, W.C. Hooper, V. Vaccarino, D.G. Harrison, and A.A. Quyyumi. 2006. The relationship between plasma levels of oxidized and reduced thiols and early atherosclerosis in healthy adults. *J Am Coll Cardiol* 47:1005–1011.

16. Ayyadevara, S., R. Alla, J.J. Thaden, and R.J. Shmookler Reis. 2007. Remarkable longevity and stress resistance of nematode P13K-null mutants. *Aging Cell* 7:13–22.

17. Baker, H. 2007. Nutrition in the elderly: Diet pitfalls and nutrition advice. *Geriatrics* 62:24–26.

18. Balch, P.A. *Prescription for Nutritional Healing.* 4th ed. Avery, 2006.

19. Balkan J., O. Kanbagli, G. Mehmetcik, U. Mutlu-Turkoglu, G. Aykac-Toker, and M. Uysal. 2003. Increased lipid peroxidation in serum and low-density lipoproteins associated with aging in humans. *Int F Vitam Nutr Res* 72:315–320.

20. Balson, P.D., K. Soderlund, B. Sjodin, and B. Ekblom. 1995. Skeletal muscle metabolism during short-duration high-intensity exercise: Influence of creatine supplementation. *Acta Physiol Scand* 154:303–310.

21. Banaclocha, M.M., A.I. Hernandez, N. Martinez, and M.L. Ferrandiz ML. 1997. N-Acetylcysteine protects against age-related increase in oxidized proteins in mouse synaptic mitochondria. *Brain Res* 762:256–258.

22. Bannai, S., and N. Tateishi. 1986. Role of membrane transport in metabolism and function of glutathione in mammals. *J Membr Biol* 89:1–8.

23. Barcelo, P., O. Wuhl, E. Servitge, A. Rousaud, C.Y. Pak. 1993. Randomized double-blind study of potassium citrate in idiopathic hypocitraturic calcium nephrolithiasis. *J Urol* 150:1761–1764.

24. Barrett, W.C., J.P. DeGnore, Y.F. Keng, Z.Y. Zhang, M.B. Yim, and P.B. Chock. 1999a. Roles of superoxide radical anion in signal transduction mediated by reversible regulation of protein-tyrosine phosphatase 1B. *J Biol Chem* 274:34543–34546.

25. Barrett, W.C., J.P. DeGnore, S. Konig, H.M. Fales, Y.F. Keng, Z.Y. Zhang, M.B. Yim, and P.B. Chock. 1999b. Regulation of PTP1B via glutathionylation of the active site cysteine 215. *Biochemistry* 38:6699–6705.

26. Barzel, U. 1995. The skeleton as an ion exchange system: implications for the role of acid-base imbalance in the genesis of osteoporosis. *J Bone Miner Res* 10:1431–1436.

27. Baumgartner, R.N., K.M. Koehler, L. Romero, and P.J. Garry. 1996. Serum albumin is associated with skeletal muscle in elderly men and women. *Am J Clin Nutr* 64:552–558.

28. Beckman, K.B., and B.N. Ames. 1998. The free radical theory of aging matures. *Physiol Rev* 78: 547–581.

29. Belin, R.J., and K. He. 2007. Magnesium physiology and pathogenic mechanisms that contribute to the development of the metabolic syndrome. *Magnes Res* 20:107–129.

30. Bergamini, E., A. Cavallini, and D.Z. Gori. 2003. The anti-ageing effects of caloric restriction may involve stimulation of macroautophagy and lysosomal degradation and can be intensified pharmacologically. *Biomed Pharmacother* 57: 203–208.

31. Bergamini, E., G. Cavallini, A. Donati, and Z. Gori. 2004. The role of macroautophagy in the ageing process, anti-ageing intervention and age-associated diseases. *Int J Biochem Cell Biol* 36:2392–2404.

32. Biolo, G., R.Y.D. Fleming, S.P. Maggi, and R.R. Wolfe. 1995. Transmembrane transport and intracellular kinetics of amino acids in human skeletal muscle. *Am J Physiol* 268:E75–E84.

33. Biolo, G., K.D. Tipton, S. Klein, and R.R. Wolfe. 1997. An abundant supply of amino acids enhances the metabolic effect of exercise on muscle protein. *Am J Physiol Endocrinol Metab* 273:E122–129.

34. Blanchetot, C., L.G. Tertoolen, and J. den Hertog. 2002. Regulation of RPTPα by oxidative stress. *EMBO J* 21:493–503.

35. Blanco, R.A., T.R. Ziegler, B.A. Carlson, P-Y Cheng, Y. Park, G.A. Cotsonis, C.J. Accardi, and D.P. Jones. 2007. Diurnal variation in glutathione and cysteine redox states in human plasma. *Am J Clin Nutr* 86:1016–1023.

36. Bohé, J., J.F. Low, R.R. Wolfe, and M.J. Rennie. 2001.

Latency and duration of stimulation of human muscle protein synthesis during continuous infusion of amino acids. *J Physiol* 532:575–579.

37. Boirie, Y., M. Dangin, P. Gachon, M-P Vasson, J-L Maubois, and B. Beaufrère. 1997a. Slow and fast dietary proteins differently moduclate postprandial protein accretion. *Proc Natl Acad Sci USA* 94:14930–14935.

38. Boirie, Y., P. Gachon, and B. Beaufrère B. 1997b. Splanchnic and whole-body leucine kinetics in young and elderly men. *Am J Clin Nutr* 65:489–495.

39. Borsheim, E., K.D. Tipton, S.E. Wolf, and R.R. Wolfe. 2002. Essential amino acids and muscle protein recovery from resistance exercise. *Am J Physiol Endocrinol Metab* 283:E648–657.

40. Bos, C., C.C. Metges, C. Gaudichon, K.J. Petzke, M.E. Pueyo, C. Morens, J. Everwand, R. Benamouzig, and D. Tomé. 2003. Postprandial kinetics of dietary amino acids are the main determinant of their metabolism after soy or milk protein ingestion in humans. *J Nutr* 133:1308–1315.

41. Brawer, J.R., R. Stein, L. Small, S. Cissé, and H.M. Schipper. 1994. Composition of gomori-positive inclusions in astrocytes of the hypothalamic arcuate nucleus. *Anat Rec* 240:407–415.

42. Breslau, N.A., L. Brinkley, K. Hill, and C.Y.C Pak. 1998. Relationship of animal protein-rich diet to kidney stone formation and calcium metabolism. *J Clin Endocrinol Metab* 66:140–146.

43. Brose, A., G. Parise, and M.A. Tarnopolsky. 2003. Creatine supplementation enhances isometric strength and body composition improvements following strength exercise training in older adults. *J Gerontol A Biol Sci Med* Sci 58:11–19.

44. Brunk, U.T., and A. Terman. 2002. The mitochondrial lysosomal axis theory of aging. Accumulation of damaged mitochondria as a result of imperfect autophagocytosis. *Eur J Biochem* 269:1996–2002.

45. Bruunsgaard, H., K. Andersen-Ranberg, J.V.B. Hjelmborg, B.K. Pedersen, and B. Jeune. 2003. Elevated levels of tumor necrosis factor-α and mortality in centenarians. *Am J Med* 115:278–283.

46. Buchner, D.M., and E.H. Wagner. 1992. Preventing frail health. *Clin Geriatr Med* 8:1.

47. Bunout, B., G. Barrera, P. de la Maza, M. Avendano, V. Gattas, M. Petermann, S. Hirsh. 2004. Effects of nutritional supplementation and resistance training on muscle strength in free living elders. Results of one-year follow. *J Nutr Health Aging* 8:68–75.

48. Burke, D.G., K. Chilibeck, S. Davison, D.G. Candow, J. Farthing, and T. Smith-Palmer. 2001. The effect of whey protein supplementation with and without creatine monohydrate combined with resistance training on lean tissue mass and muscle strength. *Int J Sport Nutr Exerc Metabol* 11:349–364.

49. Burke, D.G., P.H. Chilibeck, G. Parise, D.G. Candow, D. Mahoney, and M. Tarnopolsky. 2003. Effect of creatine and weight training on muscle creatine and performance in vegetarians. *Med Sci Sports Exerc* 35(11):1946–1955.

50. Bushinsky, D.A. 1995. Stimulated osteoclastic and suppressed osteoblastic activity in metabolic but not respiratory acidosis. *Am J Physiol* 268 (*Cell Physiol* 37):C80–C88.

51. Bushinsky, D.A. 1996. Metabolic alkalosis decreases bone calcium efflux by suppressing osteoclasts and stimulating osteoblasts. *Am J Physiol* 271 (*Renal Fluid Electrolyte Physiol* 40):F216–F222.

52. Bushinsky, D.A, and R.J. Lechleider. 1987. Mechanism of proton-induced bone calcium release: calcium carbonate dissolution. *Am J Physiol* 253 (*Renal Fluid Electrolyte Physiol* 22: F998–F1005.

53. Bushinsky, D.A., R. Levi-Setti, and F.L. Coe. 1995. Ion microprobe determination of bone surface elements: effects

of reduced medium pH. *Am J Physiol* 250 (*Renal Fluid Electrolyte Physiol* 19):F1090–F1097.

54. Bushinsky, D.A., N.S. Krieger, D.I. Geisser, E.B. Grossman, and F.L. Coe. 1983. Effects of pH on bone calcium and proton fluxes in vitro. *Am J Physiol* 245 (*Renal Fluid Electrolyte Physiol* 14) F204–F209.

55. Cai, X. 2006. Regulation of smooth muscle cells in development and vascular disease: current therapeutic strategies. *Expert Rev Cardiovasc Ther* 4:789–800.

56. Cakatay, U, A. Telci, R. Kayali, F. Tekeli, T. Akçay, and A. Sivas. 2003. Relation of aging with oxidative protein damage pramaters in rat skeletal muscle. *Clin Biochem* 36:51–55.

57. Calabrese, V, G. Scapagnini, A. Ravagna, C. Colombrita, F. Spadaro, D.A. Butterfield, and A.M. Guffrida Stella. 2004. Increased expression of heat shock proteins in rat brain during aging: relationship with mitochondrial function and glutathione redox state. *Mech Ageing Dev* 125:325–335.

58. Campbell, W.W. 2007. Synergistic use of higher-protein diets or nutritional supplements with resistance training to counter sarcopenia. *Nutrition Reviews* 65:416–422.

59. Campbell, W.W., M.C. Crim, V.R. Young, L.J. Joseph, and W.J. Evans. 1995. Effects of resistance training and dietary protein intake on protein metabolism in older adults. *Am J Physiol* 268:E1143–1153.

60. Campbell, W.W., T.A. Trappe, R.R. Wolfe, and W.J. Evans. 2001. The recommended dietary allowance for protein may not be adequate for older people to maintain skeletal muscle. *J Gerontol A Boil Sci Med Sci* 56:M373–380.

61. Candow, D.G., P.D. Chilibeck, M. Facci, S. Abeysekara, and G.A. Zello. 2006. Protein supplementation before and after resistance training in older men. *Eur J Appl Physiol* 97:548–556.

62. Carter, J.M., D.A. Bemben, A.W. Knehans, M.G. Bemben, and M.S. Witten. 2005. Does nutritional supplementation

influence adaptability of muscle to resistance training in men aged 48 to 72 years. *J Geriatr Phys Ther* 28:40–47.

63. Castillo, E.M., D. Goodman-Gruen, D. Kritz-Silverstein, D.J. Morton, and D.I. Wingard. 2003. Sarcopenia in elderly men and women: the Rancho Bernardo study. *AM J Prev Med* 25:226–231.

64. Cavallini, G., A. Donati, Z. Gori, and E. Bergamini. 2008. Towards an understanding of the anti-aging mechanism of caloric restriction. *Current Aging Science* 1:4–9.

65. Chabala, J.M., R. Levi-Setti, and D.A. Bushinsky. 1991. Alteration in surface ion composition of cultured bone during metabolic, but not respiratory, acidosis. *Am J Physiol* 261(*Renal Fluid Electrolyte Physiol* 30):F76–F84.

66. Chaput, J.P., C. Lord, M. Cloutier, M. Aubertin Leheure, E.D. Goulet, S. Rousseau, A. Khalil, and I. Dionne. 2007. Relationship between antioxidant intakes and class 1 sarcopenia in elderly men and women. *J Nutr Health Aging* 11:363–369.

67. Chen, H-Y, A.J. Lewis, P.S. Miller, and J.T. Yen. 1999. The effect of excess protein on growth performance and protein metabolism of finishing barrows and gilts. *J Anim Sci* 77:3238–3247.

68. Chen, T.S., J.P. Richie, and C.A. Lang. 1989. The effect of aging on glutathione and cysteine levels in different regions of the mouse brain. *Proc Soc Exp Biol Med* 190:399–402.

69. Chen, X., T.O. Scholl, M.J. Leskiw, M.R. Donaldson, and T.P. Stein. 2003. Association of glutathione peroxidase activity with insulin resistance and dietary fat intake during normal pregnancy. *J Clin Endocrinol Metab* 88:5963–5968.

70. Chesley, A., J.D. MacDougall, and M.A. Tarnopolsky. 1992. Changes in human muscle protein synthesis after resistance exercise. *J Appl Physiol* 73:1383–1388.

71. Chwalbinska-Moneta, J. 2003. Effect of creatine supplementation on aerobic performance and anaerobic

capacity in elite rowers in the course of endurance training. *Int J Sport Nutr Exerc Metab* 13:173–183.

72. Cicerello, E., F. Merlo, G. Gambaro, L. Maccatrozzo, A. Fandella, B. Baggio, and G. Anselmo. 1994. Effect of alkaline citrate therapy on clearance of residual renal stone fragments after extracorporeal shock wave lithotripsy in sterile calcium and infection nephrolithiasis patients. *J Urol* 151:5–9.

73. Cini, M., and A. Moretti. 1995. Studies on lipid peroxidation and protein oxidation in the aging brain. *Neurobiol Aging* 16:53–57.

74. Cocco, T., P. Sgobbo, M. Clemente, B. Lopriore, I. Grattagliano, M. Di Paola, and G. Villani. 2005. Tissue-specific changes of mitochondrial functions in aged rats: Effect of a long-term dietary treatment with N-acetylcysteine. *Free Radical Biol & Med* 38:796–805.

75. Cohen, H.Y., C. Miller, K.J. Bitterman, N.R. Wall, B. Hekking, B. Kessler, K.T. Howitz, M. Gorospe, R. de Cabo, and D.A. Sinclair. 2004. Calorie restriction promotes mammalian cell survival by inducing the SIRT1 deacetylase. *Science* 305:390–392.

76. Combaret, L., D. Dardevet, I. Rieu, M-N Pouch, D. Béchet, D. Taillandier, J. Grizard, and D. Attaix D. 2005. A leucine-supplemented diet restores the defective postprandial inhibition of proteasome-dependent proteolysis in aged rat skeletal muscle. *J Physiol* 569:489–499.

77. Committee on Military Nutrition Research (Institute of Medicine). *The Role of Protein and Amino Acids in Sustaining and Enhancing Performance.* Washington DC: National Academy Press, 1999.

78. Cooper, A.J.L. 1983. Biochemistry of sulfur-containing amino acids. *Ann Rev Biochem* 52:187–222.

79. Cooper, J.K., and C. Gardner. 1989. Effect of aging on serum albumin. *J Am Geriatric Soc* 37:1039.

80. Cordain, L., S. Boyd Eaton, A. Sebastian, N. Mann, S. Lindeberg, B.A. Watkins, J.H. O'Keefe, and J. Brand-Miller.

2005. Origins and evolution of the Western diet: health implications for the 21st century. *Am J Clin Nutr* 81:341–354.

81. Cribb, P.J., and A. Hayes. 2006. Effects of supplement timing and resistance exercise on skeletal muscle hypertrophy. *Medicine & Science in Sports & Exercise*:1918–1925.

82. Cribb, P.J., A.D. Williams, M.F. Carey, and A. Hayes. 2006. The effect of whey isolate and resistance training on strength, body composition, and plasma glutamine. *Int J Sport Nutr Exerc Metabol* 16:494–509.

83. Crowe, M.J., J.N. Weatherson, and B.F. Bowden. 2005. Effects of dietary leucine supplementation on exercise performance. *Eur J Appl Physiol* 97:664–672.

84. Cuervo, A.M., and J.F. Dice. 2000. When lysosomes get old. *Exp Gerontol* 35:119–131.

85. Cuervo, A.M., E. Bergamini, U.T. Brunk, W. Dröge, M. French, and A. Terman. 2005. Autophagy and aging. *Autophagy* 1:337–346.

86. Cummings, S.R., and L.J. Melton. 2002. Epidemiology and outcomes of osteoporotic fractures. *Lancet* 359:1761–77.

87. Curhan, G.C., W.C. Willett, E.B. Rimm, and J.J. Stampfer. 1993. A prospective study of dietary calcium and other nutrients and the risk of symptomatic kidney stones. *N Engl J Med* 328:833–838.

88. Dangin, M., Y. Boirie, C. Garcia-Rodenas, P. Gachon, J. Fauquant, P. Callier, O. Ballèvre, and B. Beaufrère. 2001. The digestion rate of protein is an independent regulating factor of postprandial protein retention. *Am J Physiol Endocrinol Metab* 280:E340–E348.

89. Dangin, M., Y. Boirie, C. Guillet, and B. Beaufrère. 2002. Influence of protein digestion rate on protein turnover in young and elderly subjects. *J Nutr* 132:3228S–3238S.

90. Dangin, M., C. Guillet, C. Garcia-Rodenas, P. Gachon, C. Bouteloup-Demange, K. Reiffers-Magnani, J. Fauquant, O. Ballèvret, and B. Beaufrère. 2003. The rate of protein

digestion affects protein gain differently during aging in humans. *J Physiol* 549:635–644.

91. Dawson-Hughes, B., and S.S. Harris. 2002. Calcium intake influences the association of protein intake with rates of bone loss in elderly men and women. *Am J Clin Nutr* 75:773–779.

92. De Cabo, R., R. Cabello, M. Rios, G. López-Lluch, D.K. Ingram, M.A. Lane, and P. Navas. 2004. Calorie restriction attenuates age-related alterations in the plasma membrane antioxidant system in rat liver. *Exp Gerontol* 39:297–304.

93. Del Roso, A., S. Vittorini, G. Cavallini, A. Donati, Z. Gori, M. Masini, M. Pollera, and E. Bergamini. 2003. Ageing-related changes in the in vivo function of rat liver macroautophagy and proteolysis. *Exp Gerontol* 38:519–527.

94. Denne, S.C., E.A. Liechty, Y.M. Liu, G. Brechtel, and A.D. Baron. 1991. Proteolysis in skeletal muscle and whole body response to euglycemic hyperinsulinemia in normal adults. *Am J Physiol* 261:E809–E814.

95. Diraison, F., P. Moulin, and M. Beylot. 2003. Contribution of hepatic de novo lipogenesis and reesterification of plasma non esterified fatty acids to plasma triglyceride synthesis during nonalcoholic fatty liver disease. *Diabetes Metab* 29:478–485.

96. Doherty, T.J. 2003. Invited review: aging and sarcopenia. J Appl Physiol 95:1717–1727.

97. Donahue, A.N., M. Aschner, L.H. Lash, T. Syversen, and W.E. Sonntag. 2006. Growth hormone administration to aged animals reduces disulfide glutathione levels in hippocampus. *Mech of Ageing & Dev* 127:57–63.

98. Donati, A., G. Cavallini, C. Paradiso, S. Vittorini, M. Pollera, Z. Gori, and E. Bergamini. 2001. Age-related changes in the autophagic proteolysis of rat isolated liver cells: Effects of anti-aging dietary restrictions. *J Gerontol A Boil Sci Med Sci* 56:B375–B383.

99. Donnelly, K.L., C.I. Smith, S.J. Schwarzenberg, J. Jessurum, M.D. Boldt, and E.J. Parks. 2005. Sources of fatty acids stored in liver and secreted via lipoproteins in patients with

nonalcoholic fatty liver disease. *J Clin Invest* 115:1343–1351.

100. Dorman, J.B., B. Albinder, T. Shroyer, and C. Kenyon. 1995. The age-1 and daf-2 genes function in a common pathway to control the life span of Caenorhabditis elegans. *Genetics* 141:1399–1406.

101. Dreyer, H.C., and E. Volpi. 2005. Role of protein and amino acids in the pathophysiology and treatment of sarcopenia. *J Am Coll Nutr* 24:140S–145S.

102. Dröge, W. 2002a. Free radicals in the physiological control of cell function. *Physiol Rev* 82:47–95.

103. Dröge, W. 2002b. Aging-related changes in the thiol/disulfide redox state: implications for the use of thiol antioxidants. *Exp Gerontol* 37:1331–1343.

104. Dröge, W. 2004. Autophagy and aging: importance of amino acid levels. *Mech Ageing Dev* 125:161–168.

105. Dröge, W., and E. Holm. 1997. Role of cysteine and glutathione in HIV infection and other diseases associated with muscle wasting and immunological dysfunction. *Fed Am Soc Exp Biol* 11:1077–1089.

106. Dröge, W., and H.M Schipper. 2007. Oxidative stress and aberrant signaling in aging and cognitive decline. *Aging Cell* 6:361–370.

107. Dröge, W., and R. Kinscherf. 2008. Aberrant insulin receptor signaling and amino acid homeostasis as a major cause of oxidative stress in aging. *Antioxid & Redox Signal* 10:661–678.

108. Dröge, W., A. Gross, V. Hack, R. Kinscherf, M. Schykowski, M. Bockstette, S. Mihm, and D. Galter. 1997. Role of cysteine and glutathione in HIV infection and cancer cachexia. Therapeutic intervention with N-acetyl-cysteine (NAC). *Advances in Pharmacol* 38:581–600.

109. Eck, H-P, C. Stahl-Hennig, G. Hunsmann, and W. Dröge. 1991. Metabolic disorder as an early consequence of simian

immunodeficiency virus infection in rhesus macaques. *Lancet* 338:346–347.

110. Elmore, S.P., T. Qian, S.F. Grissom, J.J. Lemasters. 2001. The mitochondrial permeability transition initiates autophage in rat hepatocytes. *FASEB J*:2286–2287.

111. Esmarck, B., J.L. Andersen, S. Olsen, E.A. Richter, M. Mizuno, and M. Kjaer. 2001. Timing of postexercise protein intake is important for muscle hypertrophy with resistance training in elderly humans. *J Physiol* 535:301–311.

112. Ettinger, B., C.Y. Pak, J.T. Citron, C. Thomas, B. Adams-Huet, and A. Vangessel. 1997. Potassium-magnesium citrate is an effective prophylaxis against recurrent calcium oxalate nephrolithiasis. *J Urol* 158:2069–2073.

113. Evans, W.J. 1995. What is sarcopenia? *J Gerontol A Boil Sci Med Sci* 50 (Spec No):5–8.

114. Evans, W.J. 2004. Protein nutrition, exercise and aging. *J Am Coll Nutr* 23:601S–609S.

115. Evenson, A.R., M.U. Farreed, and J.M. Menconi. 2005. GSK-3ß inhibitors reduce protein degradation in muscles from septic rats and in dexamethasone-treated myotubes. *Int J Biochem Cell Biol* 37:2226–2238.

116. Ferrante, R.J., O.A. Andreassen, B.G. Jenkins, A. Dedeoglu, S. Kuemmerle, J.K. Kubilus, R. Daddurah-Daouk, S.M. Hersch, and M.F. Beal. 2000. Neuroprotective effects of creatine in a transgenic mouse model of Huntington's disease. *J Neurosci* 20:4389–4397.

117. Fiatarone, M.A., E.C. Marks, N.D. Ryan, C.N. Meredith, L.A. Lipsitz, and W.J. Evans. 1990. High-intensity strength training in nonagenarians. Effects on skeletal muscle. *JAMA* 13:3029–3034.

118. Fiatarone, M.A., E.F. O'Neill, N.D. Ryan, K.M. Clements, G.R. Solares, M.E. Nelson, S.B. Roberts, J.J. Kehayias, L.A. Lipsitz, and W.J. Evans. 1994. Exercise training and nutritional supplementation for physical frailty in very elderly people. *N Engl J Med* 330:1769–1775.

119. Fischer, E.H., H. Charbonneau, and N.K. Tonks. 1991. Protein tyrosine phosphatases: A diverse family of intracellular and transmembrane enzymes. *Science* 253:401–406.

120. Flagg, E.W., R.J. Coates, D.P. Jones, J.W. Eley, E.W. Gunter, B. Jackson, and R.S. Greenberg. 1993. Plasma total glutathione in humans and its association with demographic and health-related factors. *British Journal of Nutrition* 70:797–808.

121. Fraga, C.G., M.K. Shigenaga, J.W. Park, P. Degan, and B.N. Ames. 1990. Oxidative damage to DNA during aging: 8-hydroxy-2'-deoxyguanosine in rat organ DNA and urine. *Proc Natl Acad Sci USA* 87:4533–4537.

122. Frank, J.W., J. Escobar, A. Suryawan, S.R. Kimball, H.V. Nguyen, S. Leonard, and T.A. Davis. 2005. Protein synthesis and translation initiation factor activation in neonatal pigs fed increasing levels of dietary protein. *J Nutr*:1374–1381.

123. Frassetto, L., and A. Sebastian. 1996. Age and systemic acid-base equilibrium: analysis of published data. *J Gerontol* 51A:B91–B99.

124. Frassetto, L., R.C. Morris Jr., and A. Sebastian. 1996. Effect of age on blood acid-base composition in humans: role of age-related renal functional decline. *Am J Physiol* 271:1114–1122.

125. Frassetto, L., R.C. Morris Jr., and A. Sebastian. 1997. Potassium bicarbonate reduces urinary nitrogen excretion in postmenopausal women. *J Clin Endrocrinol Metab* 82:254–259.

126. Frassetto, L., K.M. Todd, R.C. Morris Jr., and A. Sebastian. 2000. Worldwide incidence of hip fracture in elderly women. *J Gerontol Series A: Biological Sciences and Medical Sciences* 55:M585–M592.

127. Frassetto, L., R.C. Morris Jr., and A. Sebastian. 2005. Long-term persistence of the urine calcium-lowering effect of potassium bicarbonate in postmenopausal women. *J Clin Endocrinol Metab* 90:831–834.

128. Frestedt, J.L., J.L. Zenk, M.A. Kuskowski, L.S Ward,

and E.D. Bastian. 2008. A whey-protein supplement increases fat loss and spares lean muscle in obese subjects: a randomized human clinical study. *Nutrition & Metabolism* 5:8 doi:10.1186/1743-7075-5-8.

129. Freyssenet, D., P. Berthon, C. Denis, J.C. Barthelemy, C.Y. Guezennec, and J.C. Chatard. 1996. Effect of a 6-week endurance training programme and branched-chain amino acid supplementation on histomorphometric characteristics of aged human muscle. *Arch Physiol Biochem* 104:157–162.

130. Frontera, W.R., C.N. Meredith, K.P. O'Reilly, H.G. Knuttgen, and W.J. Evans. 1988. Strength conditioning in older men: skeletal muscle hypertrophy and improved function. *J Appl Physiol* 64:1038–1044.

131. Fukagawa, N.K., K.L. Minaker, V.R. Young, D.E. Matthews, D.M. Bier, and J.W. Rowe. 1989. Leucine metabolism in aging humans: effect of insulin and substrate availability. *Am J Physiol* 256: E288–E294.

132. Furukawa, T., S.N. Meydani, and J.B. Blumberg. 1987. Reversal of age-associated decline in immune responsiveness by dietary glutathione supplementation in mice. *Mech Ageing Dev* 38: 107–117.

133. Gelfand, R.A., and E.J. Barrett. 1987. Effect of physiological hyperinsulinemia on skeletal muscle protein synthesis and breakdown in man. *J Clin Invest* 80:1–6.

134. Glaumann, H., J.L. Ericsson, and L. Marzella. 1981. Mechanisms of intralysosomal degradation with special reference to autophagocytosis of cell organelles. *Int Rev Cytol* 73:149–182.

135. Glauser, A., W. Hochreiter, P. Jaeger, and B. Hess. 2000. Determinants of urinary excretion of Tamm-Horsfall protein in non-selected kidney stone formers and healthy subjects. *Nephrol Dial Transplant* 15:1580–1587.

136. Goldhaber, P., and H. Rabadjija. 1987. H$^+$ stimulation of cell-mediated bone resorption in tissue culture. *Am J Physiol* 253 (*Endocrinol Metab* 16):E90–E98.

137. Goldstein, B.J., K. Mahadev, W. Xiangdong, L. Zhu, and H. Motoshima. 2005. Role of insulin-induced reactive oxygen species in the insulin signaling pathway. *Antioxidants & Redox Signaling* 7:1021–1031.

138. Griendling, K.K., and R.W. Alexander. 1997. Oxidative stress and cardiovascular disease. *Circulation* 96:3264–3275.

139. Gross, A., V. Hack, C. Stahl-Hemming, and W. Dröge. 1996. Elevated hepatic γ-glutamyl cysteine synthetase (δ-GCS) activity and abnormal sulfate levels in liver and muscle tissue may explain abnormal cysteine and glutathione levels in SIV-infected rhesus macaques. *AIDS Res and Human Retrovir* 12:1639–1641.

140. Gupta, A., M. Hasan, R. Chander, and N.K. Kapoor. 1991. Age-related elevation of lipid peroxidation products: diminution of superoxide dismutase activity in the central nervous system of rats. *Gerontology* 37: 305–309.

141. Hack, V., A. Gross, R. Kinscherf, M. Bockstette, W. Fiers, G. Berke, and W. Dröge. 1996. Abnormal glutathione and sulfate levels after interleukin-6 treatment and in tumor-induced cachexia. *FASEB J* 10:1219–1226.

142. Hack, V., R. Breitkreutz, R. Kinscherf, H. Röhrer, P. Bartsch, F. Taut, A. Benner, and W. Dröge W. 1998. The redox state as a correlate of senescence and wasting and as a target for therapeutic intervention. *Blood* 92:59–67.

143. Halperin, M.L., and R.L. Jungas. 1983. Metabolic production and renal disposal of hydrogen ions. *Kidney Int* 24:709–713.

144. Hamadeh, M.J., and J.L. Hoffer. 2001. Use of sulfate production as a measure of short-term sulfur amino acid catabolism in humans. *Am J Physiol Endrocrinol Metab* 280:E857–E866.

145. Hamilton, M.L., H. Van Remmen, J.A. Drake, H. Yang, Z.M. Guo, K. Kewitt, C.A. Walter, and A. Richardson. 2001. Does oxidative damage to DNA increase with age? *Proc Natl Acad Sci* 98:10469–10474.

146. Hamm, L.L., and R.J. Alpern. "Regulation of Acid-Base

balance, Citrate, and Urine Ph." In *Kidney Stones: Medical and Surgical Management*, edited by F.L. Coe, M.J. Favus, C.Y.C. Pak, J.H. Parks, and G.M. Preminger, 289–302. Philadelphia: Lippincott-Raven, 1996.

147. Hara, T., K. Nakamura, M. Matsui, A. Yamamoto, Y. Nakahara, R. Suzuki-Migishima, M. Yokoyama, K. Mishima, I. Saito, H. Okano, and N. Mizushima. 2006. Suppression of basal autophagy in neural cells causes neurodegenerative disease in mice. *Nature* 441, 885–889.

148. Harman, D. 1956. Aging: a theory based on free radical and radiation chemistry. *J Gerontol* 11: 298–300.

149. Harman, D. 1981. The aging process. *Proc Natl Acad Sc USA* 78:7124–7128.

150. Hars, E.S., H. Qi, A.G. Ryazanov, S. Jin, L. Cai, C. Hu, and L.F. Liu. 2007. Autophagy regulates ageing in *C. elegans*. *Autophagy* 3:93–95.

151. Hasselgren, P.O., M.J. Menconi, and M.U. Fareed. 2005. Novel aspects on the regulation of muscle wasting in sepsis. *Int J Biochem Cell Biol* 37:2156–2168.

152. Hauer, K., Hildebrandt, W. Sehl, L. Edler, P. Oster, and W. Dröge. 2003. Improvement in muscular performance and decrease in tumor necrosis factor level in old age after antioxidant treatment. *J Mol Med* 81:118–125.

153. Heaney, R.P., K. Rafferty, and M. Davies. 2005. Letters to the Editor. *J Clin Endocrinol & Metab* 90(7):4417–4420.

154. Hespel, P., B. Op't Eijnde, M. Van Leemputte, B. Urs⊠, P.L. Greehaff, V. Labarque, S. Dymarkowski, P. Van Hecke, and E.A. Richter. 2001. Oral creatine supplementation facilitates the rehabilitation of disuse atrophy and alters the expression of muscle myogenic factors in humans. *J Physiol (Lond)* 536:625–633.

155. Hess, B., S. Jordi, L. Zipperle, E. Ettinger, and R. Giovanoli. 2000. Citrate determines calcium oxalate crystallization kinetics and crystal morphology: studies in the presence of Tamm-Horsfall protein of a healthy subject and a severely

recurrent calcium stone former. *Nephrol Dial Transplant* 15:366–374.

156. Hess, B. 2006. Acid-base metabolism: implications for kidney stone formation. *Urol Res* 34:134–138.

157. Hildebrandt, W., S. Alexander, P. Bärtsch, and W. Dröge. 2002a. Effect of N-acetyl-cysteine on the hypoxic ventilatory response and erythropoietin production: linkage between plasma thiol redox state and O_2 chemosensitivity. *Blood* 99:1552–1555.

158. Hildebrandt, W., R. Kinscherf, K. Hauer, E. Holm, and W. Dröge. 2002b. Plasma cystine concentration and redox state in aging and physical exercise. *Mech of Ageing and Dev* 123: 1269–1281.

159. Hildebrandt, W., A. Hamann, H. Krakowski-Roosen, R. Kinscherf, K. Dugi, R. Sauer, S. Lacher, N. Nöbel, A. Bodens, V. Bellou, L. Edler, P. Nawroth, and W. Dröge. 2004. Effect of thiol antioxidant on body fat and insulin reactivity. *J Mol Med* 82:336–344.

160. Hirota, K., T. Hara, S. Hosoi, Y. Sasaki, Y. Hara, and T. Adachi. 2005. Two cases of hyperkalemia after administration of hypertonic mannitol during craniotomy. *J Anesth* 19:75–77.

161. Hoffman, J., N. Ratamess, J. Kang, G. Mangine, A. Faigenbaum, and J. Stout. 2006. Effect of creatine and beta-alanine supplementation on performance and endocrine responses in strength/power athletes. *Int J Sport Nutr Exerc Metab* 16:430–446.

162. Honda, Y., and S. Honda. 1999. The daf-2 gene network for longevity regulates oxidative stress resistance and Mn-superoxide dismutase gene expression in *Caenorhabditis elegans*. *Faseb J* 13:1385–1393.

163. Hubbard, S.R. 1997. Crystal structure of the activated insulin receptor tyrosine kinase in complex with peptide substrate and ATP analog. *EMBO J* 16:5572–5581.

164. Huso, M.E., J.S. Hampl, C.S. Johnston, and P.D. Swan. 2002.

Creatine supplementation influences substrate utilization at rest. *J Appl Physiol* 93:2018–2022.

165. Hwangbo, D.S., B. Gershman, M.P. Tu, M. Palmer, and M. Tatar M. 2004. *Drosophila* dFOXO controls life span and regulates insulin signaling in brain and fat body. *Nature* 429:562–566.

166. Inal, M.E., G. Kanbak, and E. Sunal. 2001. Antioxidant enzyme activities and malondialdehyde levels related to aging. *Clin Chim Acta* 305:75–80.

167. Ivanovski, O., D. Szumilak, T. Nguyen-Khoa, N. Ruellan, O. Phan, B. Lacour, B. Descamps-Latscha, T.B. Drüeke, and Z.A. Massy. 2005. The antioxidant N-acetylcysteine prevents accelerated atherosclerosis in uremic apolipoprotein E knockout mice. *Kidney Int* 67: 2288–2294.

168. Jackson, R.D., A.Z. LaCroix, M. Gass, and others. 2006. Calcium plus vitamin D supplementation and the risk of fractures. *N Engl J Med* 354:669–83. (Erratum, *N Engl J Med* 354:1102.)

169. Jaeschke, H., and A. Wendel. 1985. Diurnal fluctuation and pharmacological alternation of mouse organ glutathione content. *Biochemical Pharmacology* 34:1029–1033.

170. Janssen, I., D.S. Shepard, P.T. Katzmarzyk, and R. Roubenoff. 2004. The health care costs of sarcopenia in the United States. *J Am Geriatr Soc* 52:80–85.

171. Jasminka, Z., R.D. Ilich PhD, and R.D. Kerstetter PhD. 2000. Nutrition in bone health revisited: a story beyond calcium. *J Am Col Ntr* 19:6,715–737.

172. Johnston Jr, C.C. 1996. Development of clinical practice guidelines for prevention and treatment of osteoporosis. *Calcif Tissue Int* 59 (Suppl 1):S30–33.

173. Jones, D.P., V.C. Mody Jr, J.L. Carlson, M.J. Lynn, and P. Sternberg Jr. 2002. Redox analysis of human plasma allows separation of pro-oxidant events of aging from decline in antioxidant defenses. *Free Rad Biol & Med* 33:1290–1300.

174. Jones, D.P. 2006a. Extracellular redox state: refining the

definition of oxidative stress in aging. *Rejuvenation Research* 9:169–181.

175. Jones, D.P. 2006b. Redefining oxidative stress. *Antioxidants & Redox Signaling* 8:1865–1879.

176. Kanis, J.A., L.J. Melton 3rd, C. Christiansen, C.C. Johnston, and N. Khaltaev. 1994. The diagnosis of osteoporosis. *J Bone Miner Res* 9:1137–1141.

177. Kapahi, P., M.E. Boulton, and T.B. Kirkwood. 1999. Positive correlation between mammalian life span and cellular resistance to stress. *Free Radic Biol Med* 26:495–500.

178. Kapahi, P., B.M. Zid, T. Harper, D. Koslover, V. Sapin, and S. Benzer. 2004. Regulation of life span in *Drosophila* by modulation of genes in the TOR signaling pathway. *Curr Biol* 14:885–890.

179. Kasapoglu, M., and T. Azben. 2001. Alterations of antioxidant enzymes and oxidative stress markers in aging. *Exp Gerontol* 36:209–220.

180. Katsanos, C.S., H. Kobayashi, M. Sheffield-Moore M, and others. 2006. A high proportion of leucine is required for optimal stimulation of the rate of muscle protein synthesis by essential amino acids in the elderly. *Am J Physiol Endocrinol Metab* 291:E381–387.

181. Kenyon, C., J. Chang, E. Gensch, A. Rudner, and R. Tabtiang. 1993. *C. elegans* mutant that lives twice as long as wild type. *Nature* 366:461–464.

182. Kerr, B.J., and R.A. Easter. 1995. Effect of feeding reduced protein amino acid-supplemented diets on nitrogen and energy balance in grower pigs. *J Anim Sci* 73:3000–3008.

183. Kerr, B.J., J.T. Yen, J.A. Nienaber, and R.A. Easter. 2003. Influences of dietary protein level, amino acid supplementation and environmental temperatures on performance, body composition, organ weights and total heat production of growing pigs. *J Anim Sci* 81:1998–2007.

184. Kerstetter, J.E., K.O. O'Brien, and K.L. Insogna. 2003.

Dietary protein calcium metabolism, and skeletal homeostasis revisited. *Am J Clin Nutr* 78(suppl):584S–92S.

185. Kerstetter, J.E., K.O. O'Brien, D.M. Caseria, D.E. Wall, and K.L. Insogna. 2005. The impact of dietary protein on calcium absorption and inetic measures of bone turnover in women. *J Clin Endocrinol Metab* 90:26–31.

186. Kim, J., and D.J. Klionsky. 2000. Authophagy, cytoplasm-to-vacuole targeting pathway, and pexophagy in yeast and mammalian cells. *Annu rev Biochem* 69:303–342.

187. Kimball, S.R., P. Farrell, and L.S. Jefferson. 2002. Exercise effects on muscle insulin signaling and action invited review: role of insulin in translational control of protein synthesis in skeletal muscle by amino acids or exercise. *J Appl Physiol* 93:1168–1180.

188. Kimball, S.R., and L.S. Jefferson. 2004. Regulation of global and specific mRNA translation by oral administration of branched-chain amino acids. *Biochem Biophys Res Commun* 313:423–427.

189. Kimura, K.D., H.A. Tissenbaum, Y. Liu, and G. Ruvkun G. 1997. Daf-2, an insulin receptor-like gene that regulates longevity and diapause in *Caenorhabditis elegans*. *Science* 277:942–946.

190. Kinscherf, R., V. Hack, T. Fischbach, B. Friedmann, C. Weiss, L. Edler, P. Bartsch, and W. Dröge. 1996. Low plasma glutamine in combination with high glutamate levels indicate risk for loss of body cell mass in healthy individuals: the effect of N-acetylcysteine. *J Mol Med* 74: 393–400.

191. Kjellmer, I. 1965. The potassium ion as a vasodilator during muscular exercise. *Acta Physiol Scand* 63:460–468.

192. Klionsky, D.J., and S.D. Emr. 2000. Autophagy as a regulated pathway of cellular degradation. *Science* 290:1717–1721.

193. Komatsu, M., S. Waguri, T. Chiba, S. Murata, J. Iwata, I. Tanida, T. Ueno, Y. Koike Muchiyama, E. Kominami, and K. Tanaka. 2006. Loss of autophagy in the central nervous

system causes neurodegeneration in mice. *Nature* 441:880–884.

194. Koopman, R., L. Verdijk, R.J.F. Manders, A.P. Gijsen, M. Gorselink, E. Pijpers, A.J.M. Wagenmakers, and L.J.C. van Loon. 2006. Co-ingestion of protein and leucine stimulates muscle protein synthesis rates to the same extent in young and elderly lean men. *Am J Clin Nutr* 84:623–632.

195. Koopman, R., W.H.M. Saris, A.J.M. Wagenmakers, and L.J.C. van Loon. 2007. Nutritional interventions to promote post-exercise muscle protein synthesis. *Sports Med* 37:896–906.

196. Kops, G.J., T.B. Dansen, P.D. Polderman, I. Saarloos, K.W. Wirtz, P.J. Coffer, T.T. Huajg, J.L. Bos, R.H. Medema, and B.M. Burgering. 2002. Forkhead transcription factor FOXO3a protects quiescent cells from oxidative stress. *Nature* 419:316–321.

197. Krebs, M., M. Krssak, E. Bernroider, C. Anderwald, A. Brehm, M. Meyerspeer, P. Nowotny, E. Roth, W. Waldhausl, and M. Roden. 2002. Mechanism of amino acid-induced skeletal muscle insulin resistance in humans. *Diabetes* 51:599–605.

198. Krieger, N.S., N.E. Sessler, and D.A. Bushinsky. 1992. Acidosis inhibits osteoblastic and stimulates osteoclastic activity in vitro. *Am J Physiol* 262 (*Renal Fluid Electrolyte Physiol*) 31:F442–F448.

199. Krishna, G.C., and S.C. Kapoor. 1991. Potassium depletion exacerbates essential hypertension. *Ann Intern Med* 15:77–83.

200. Kumaran, S., B. Deepak, B. Naveen, and C. Panneerselvam. 2003. Effects of levocarnitine on mitochondrial antioxidant systemes and oxidative stress in aged rats. *Drugs R&D* 4: 141–147.

201. Kurtz, I., T. Maher, H.N. Hulter, M. Schambelan, and A. Sebastian. 1983. Effect of diet on plasma acid-base composition in normal humans. *Kidney Int* 24:670–680.

202. Lands, L.C., V.L. Grey, and A.A. Smountas. 1999. Effect of supplementation with a cysteine donor on muscular performance. *J Appl Physiol* 87:1381–1385.

203. Larsson, L., G. Grimby, and J. Karlsson. 1979. Muscle strength and speed of movement in relation to age and muscle morphology. *J Appl Physiol* 46:451–456.

204. Lee, J.I., M. Londono, L.L. Hirschberger, and M.H. Stipanuk. 2004. Regulation of cysteine dioxygenase and gamma-glutamylcysteine synthetase is associated with hepatic cysteine level. J Nutr Biochem 15(2):112–122.

205. Lemann Jr., J. "Pathogenesis of Idiopathic Hypercalciuria and Nephrolithiasis." In *Disorders of Bone and Mineral Metabolism*, edited by F.L. Coe and M.J. Favus, 685–706. New York: Raven Press, 1992.

206. Lemann Jr., J. "Calcium and Phosphate Metabolism: An Overview in Health and in Calcium Stone Formers." In *Kidney Stones: Medical and Surgical Management*, edited by F.L. Coe, M.J. Favus, C.Y.C. Pack, J.H. Parks, and G.M. Preminger, 259–288. Philadelphia: Lippincott-Raven, 1996.

207. Lemann Jr., J. 1999. Relationship between urinary calcium and net acid excretion as determined by dietary protein and potassium: a review. *Nephron* 81 (Suppl 1):18–25.

208. Lemann Jr., J., and J.R. Litzow, and E.J. Lennon. 1966. The effects of chronic acid loads in normal man: further evidnece for the participation of bone mineral in the defense against chronic metabolic acidosis. *J clin Invest* 45:1608–1614.

209. Lemann Jr., J., J.R. Litzow, and E.J. Lennon. 1967. Studies of the mechanism by which chronic metabolic acidosis augments urinary calcium excretion in man. *J Clin Invest* 46:1318–1328.

210. Lemann Jr., J., R.W. Gray, and J.A. Pleuss. 1989. Potassium bicarbonate, but no sodium bicarbonate, reduces urinary calcium excretion and improves calcium balance in healthy men. *Kidney Int* 35:688–695.

211. Lemann Jr., J., D.A. Bushinsky, and L. Lee Hamm. 2003.

Bone buffering of acid and base in humans. *Am J Physiol Renal Physiol* 285:F811–F832.

212. Lennon, E.J., J. Lemann Jr., and J.R. Litzow. 1966. The effect of diet and stool composition on the net external acid balance of normal subjects. *J Clin Invest* 45:1601–1607.

213. Lentner, C. *Geigy Scientific Tables.* 8th ed. Vol. 1, *Units of Measurement, Body Fluids, Composition of the Body, Nutrition.* West Caldwell, N.J.: Ciba-Geigy Corporation, 1981.

214. Levine, B., and D.J. Klionsky. 2004. Development by self-digestion: molecular mechanisms and biological functions of autophagy. *Dev Cell* 6:463–477.

215. Levine, R.L., and E.R. Stadtman. 2001. Oxidative modification of proteins during aging. *Exp Gerontol* 36:1495–1502.

216. Li, B.G., P.O. Hasselgren, and C.H. Fang. 2005. Insulin-like growth factor-1 inhibits dexamethasone-induced proteolysis in cultured L6 myotubes through P13K/Akt/GSK-3ß and P13K/AktmTOR-dependent mechanisms. *Int J Biochem Cell Biol* 37: 2207–2216.

217. Li, M., J-F Chiu, B.T. Mossman, and N.K. Fukagawa. 2006. Downregulation of manganese-superoxide dismutase through phosphorylation of FOXO3a by Akt in explanted vascular smooth muscle cells from old rats. *J Biol Chem* 281: 40429–40439.

218. Li, X., B. Monks, Q. Ge, and M.J. Birnbaum. 2007. Akt/PKB regulates hepatic metabolism by directly inhibiting PGC-1⊠ transcription coactivator. *Nature* 447:1012–1016.

219. Liang, H., E.J. Masoro, J.F. Nelson, R. Strong, C.A. McMahan, and A. Richardson. 2003. Genetic mouse models of extended life span. *Exp Gerontol* 38:1353–1364.

220. Lin, J., C. Handschin, and B. Spiegelman. 2005. Metabolic control through the PGC-1 family of transcription coactivators. *Cell Metabolism* 1:361–370.

221. Lin, Y.J., L. Seroude, and S. Benzer. 1998. Extended life span

and stress resistance in the *Drosophila* mutant *methuselah*. *Science* 282: 943–946.

222. Linnane, A.W., S. Marzuki, T. Ozawa, and M. Tanaka. 1989. Mitochondrial DNA mutations as an important contributor to ageing and degenerative diseases. *Lancet* 25:642–645.

223. Lopez, J., R.D. Goodband, G.L. Allee, G.W. Jesse, L.J. Nelssen, M.D. Tokach, D. Spiers, and B.A. Becker. 1994. The effects of diets formulated on an ideal protein basis on growth performance, carcass characteristics, and thermal balance of finishing gilts housed in a hot, diurnal environment. *J Anim Sci* 72:367–379.

224. Lord, C., J.P. Chapuut, M. Aubertin-Leheure, M. Labonté, and I.J. Dionne. 2007. Dietary animal protein intake: association with muscle mass index in older women. *J Nutr Health Aging* 11:383–387.

225. Lucas, D.T., and L.I. Szweda. 1998. Cardiac reperfusion injury: aging, lipid peroxidation, and mitochondrial dysfunction. *Proc Natl Acad USA* 95:510–514.

226. Lutz, J. 1984. Calcium balance and acid-base status of women as affected by increased protein intake and by sodium bicarbonate ingestion. *Am J Clin Nutr* 39:281–288.

227. Macdonald, H.M., S.A. New, M.H.N. Golden, M.K. Campbell, and D.M. Reid. 2004. Nutritional associations with bone loss during the menopausal transition: evidence of a beneficial effect of calcium, alcohol, and fruits and vegetable nutrients and of a detrimental effect of fatty acids. *Am J Clin Nutr* 79:155–165.

228. Macdonald, H.M., S.A. New, W.D. Fraser, M.K. Campbell, and D.M. Reid. 2005. Low dietary potassium intakes and high dietary estimates of net endogenous acid production are associated with low bone mineral density in premenopausal women and increased markers of bone resorption in postmenopausal women. *Am J Clin Nutr* 81 (No. 4):923–933.

229. MacDougall, J.D., M.A. Tarnopolsky, A. Chesley, and

S.A. Atkinson. 1992. Changes in muscle protein synthesis following heavy resistance exercise in humans: a pilot study. *Acta Physiol Scand* 146:403–404.

230. MacDougall, J.D., M.J. Gibala, M.A. Tarnopolsky, J.R. MacDonald, S.A. Interisano, and K.E. Yarasheski. 1995. The time course for elevated muscle protein synthesis following heavy resistance exercise. *Can J Appl Physiol* 20:480–486.

231. Magee, E.A., C.J. Richardson, R. Hughes, and J.H. Cummings. 2000. Contribution of dietary protein to sulfide production in the large intestine: an in vitro and a controlled feeding study in humans. *Am J Clin Nutr* 72:1488–1494.

232. Mammucari, C., G. Milan, V. Romanello, E. Masiero, R. Rudolf, P. Del Piccolo, S.J. Burden, R. Di Lisi, C. Sandri, J. Zhao, A.L. Goldberg, S. Schiaffino, and M. Sandri. 2007. FoxO3 controls autophagy in skeletal muscle in vivo. *Cell Metabolism* 6: 458–471.

233. Marangella, M., N.M. De Stefano, S. Casalis, S. Berutti, P.D. Amelio, and G.C. Isaia. 2004. Effects of potassium citrate supplementation on bone metabolism. 74:330–335.

234. Marangella, M. "Hyperuricemic Syndromes: Pathophysiology and Therapy." In *Hyperuricemic Syndromes: Pathophysiology and Therapy*, edited by C. Ronco and F. Rodeghiero, 132–148C. Basel, Karger, 147, 2005.

235. Martinez, M., A.I. Hermandez, and N. Martinez. 2000. N-acetylcysteine delays age-associated memory impairment in mice: role in synaptic mitochondria. *Brain Res* 855, 100–106.

236. Marzabadi, M.R., R.S Sohal, and U.T. Brunk. 1991. Mechanisms of lipofuscinogenesis: effect of the inhibition of lysosomal proteinases and lipases under varying concentrations of ambient oxygen in cultured rat neonatal myocardial cells. *APMIS* 99:416–426.

237. Matheu, A., A. Maraver, P. Klatt, I. Flores, I. Garcia-Cao, C. Borras, J.M. Flores, J. Vina, M.A. Blasco, and M. Serrano.

2007. Delayed ageing through damage protection by the Arf/p53 pathway. Nature 448:375–379.

238. Matthews, D.E. 1999. "Proteins and Amino Acids." In *Modern Nutrition in Health and Disease*, edited by M.E. Shils, 11–48. Baltimore: Williams & Wilkins, 1999.

239. Maurer, M., W. Riesen, J. Muser, H.N. Hulter, and R. Krapf. 2002. Neutralization of Western diet inhibits bone resoption independently of K intake and reduces cortisol secretion in humans. *Am J Physiol Renal Physiol* 284:F32–F40.

240. May, R.C., R.A. Kelly, and W.E. Mitch. 1986. Metabolic acidosis stimulates protein degradation in rat muscle by a glucocorticoid-dependent mechanism. *J Clin Invest* 77:614–621.

241. McClung, J.P., C.A. Roneker, W. Mu, D.J. Lisk, P. Langlais, F. Liu, and X.G. Lei. 2004. Development of insulin resistance and obesity in mice overexpressing cellular glutathione peroxidase. *Proc Natl Acad Sci USA* 101:8852–8857.

242. McKenzie, D., E. Bua, S. McKiernan, Z. Cao, J. Wanagat, and J.M. Aiken. 2002. Mitochondrial DNA deletion mutations. A causal role in sarcopenia. *Eur J Biochem* 269:2010–2015.

243. Meister, A., and M.E. Anderson. 1983. Glutathione. *Annu Rev Biochem* 52:711–760.

244. Melendez, A., Z. Talloczy, M. Seaman, E.L. Eskelinen, D.H. Hall, and B. Levine. 2003. Autophage genes are essential for dauer development and life span extension in *C.elegans*. *Science* 301:1387–1391.

245. Melov, S., M.A. Tarnopolsky, K. Beckman, K. Felkey, and A. Hubbard. 2007. Resistance exercise reverses aging in human skeletal muscle. 23:e465.

246. Melton 3rd, L.J., S. Khosla, C.S. Crowson, M.K. O'Connor, and W.M. O'Fallon. 2000. Epidemiology of sarcopenia. *J Am Geriatr Soc* 48:625–630.

247. Meredith, C.N., W.R. Frontera, K.P. O'Reilly, and W.J. Evans. 1992. Body composition in elderly men: effect of

dietary modification during strength training. *J Am Geriatr Soc* 40:155–162.

248. Migliaccio, E., M. Giorgio, S. Mele, G. Pelicci, P. Reboldi, P.P. Pandolfi, L. Lanfrancone, and P.G. Pelicci. 1999. The p66[shc] adaptor protein controls oxidative stress response and life span in mammals. *Nature* 402:309–313.

249. Miller, S.L., K.D. Tipton, D.L. Chinkes, S.E. Wolf, and R.R. Wolfe. 2003. Independent and combined effects of amino acids and glucose after resistance exercise. *Med Sci Sports Exerc* 35:449–455.

250. Miquel, J., P.R. Lundgren, and J.E. Johnson. 1978. Spectrophotofluorometric and electron microscopic study of lipofuscin accumulation in the testis of aging mice. *J Gerontol* 33:5–19.

251. Miquel, J., M.L. Ferrandiz, E. De Juan, I. Sevila, and M. Martinez. 1995. N-acetylcysteine protects against age-related decline of oxidative phosphorylation in liver mitochrondria. *Eur J Pharmacol* 292:333–335.

252. Mitch, W.E., and H. Robert. 1998. Mechanisms causing loss of lean body mass in kidney disease. *Am J Clin Nutr* 67:359–366.

253. Monk, R.D., and D.A. Bushinsky. "Pathogenesis of Idiopathic Hypercalciuria." In *Kidney Stones: Medical and Surgical Management*, edited by F.L. Coe, M.J. Favus, C.Y.C Pak, J.H. Parks, and G.M. Preminger, 759–772, Philadelphia: Lippincott-Raven, 1996.

254. Mörck, C., and M. Pilon. 2007. Caloric restriction and autophagy in *Caenorhabditis elegans*. *Autophagy* 3:51–53.

255. Morris, J.Z., H.A. Tissenbaum, and G. Ruvkun. 1996. A phosphatidylinositol-3 OH kinase family member regulating longevity and diapause in *Caenorhabditis elegans*. *Nature* 382:536–539.

256. Morris Jr., R.C., and A. Sebastian. 2002. Alkali therapy in renal tubular acidosis: who needs it? *J Am Soc Nephrol* 13:2186–2188.

257. Mortimore, G.E., and A.R. Pösö. 1987. Intracellular protein catabolism and its control during nutrient deprivation and supply. *Ann Rev Nutr* 7:539–564.

258. Murray, C.A., and M.A. Lynch. 1998. Evidence that increased hippocampal expression of the cytokine interleukin-1 ☒ is a common trigger for age- and stress-induced impairments in long-term potentiation. *J Neurosci* 18:2974–2981.

259. Muscari, C., C.M. Caldarera, and C. Guarnieri. 1990. Age-dependent production of mitochondrial hydrogen peroxide, lipid peroxides and fluorescent pigments in the rat heart. *Basic Res Cardiol* 85:172–178.

260. Naber, T.H.J., A. de Bree, T.R.J. Schermer, J. Bakkeren, B. Bar, G. de Wild, and M.B. Katan. 1997. Specificity of indexes of malnutrition when applied to apparently healthy people: The effect of age. *Am J Clin Nutr* 65:1721.

261. Nadler, J., T. Buchanan, R. Natarajan, I. Antoipillai, R. Bergman, and R. Rude. 1993. Magnesium deficiency produces insulin resistance and increased thromboxane synthesis. *Hypertension* 21:1024–1029.

262. National Osteoporosis Foundation. 1998. Osteoporosis: review of the evidence for prevention, diagnosis, and treatment and cost-effectiveness analysis. *Osteoporos Int* 8(suppl):S1–88.

263. Neuman, R.B., H.L. Bloom, I. Shukrullah, L.A. Darrow, D. Kleinbaum, D.P. Jones, and S.C. Dudley Jr. 2007. Oxidative stress markers are associated with persistent atrial fibrillation. *Clin Chem* 53:1652–1657.

264. New, S.A., H.M. MacDonald, M.K. Campbell, J.C. Martin, M.J. Garton, S.P. Robins, and D.M. Reid. 2004. Lower estimates of net endogenous noncarbonic acid production are positively associated with indexes of bone health in premenopausal and perimenopausal women. *Am J Clin Nutr* 79:131–138.

265. Nixon, R.A., J. Wegiel, A. Kumar, W.H. Yu, C. Peterhoff, A. Cataldo, and A.M. Cuervo. 2005. Extensive involvement

of autophagy in Alzheimer disease: An immuno-electron microscopy study. *J of Neuropathology & Exp Neurology* 64:113–122.

266. O'Donnell, E., and M.A. Lynch. 1998. Dietary antioxidant supplementation reverses age-related neuronal changes. *Neurobiol Aging* 19:461–467.

267. Ohsumi, Y. 2001. Molecular dissection of autophagy: two ubiquitin-like systems. *Nature Rev Mol Cell Biol* 2:211–216.

268. Orlandi, A., M.L. Bochaton-Piallat, G. Gabbiani, and L.G. Spagnoll. 2006. Aging, smooth muscle cells and vascular pathobiology: implications for atherosclerosis. *Atherosclerosis* 188:221–230.

269. Orr, W.C., and R.S. Sohal. 1994. Extension of life span by overexpression of superoxide dismutase and catalase in *Drosophila melanogaster*. *Science* 263:1128–1130.

270. Osorio, A.V., and U.S. Alon. 1997. The relationship between urinary calcium, sodium, and potassium excretion and the role of potassium in treating idiopathic hypercalciuria. *Pediatrics* 100:675–681.

271. Otten, J.J., J. Pitzi Hellwig, and L.D. Meyers. *Dietary Reference Intakes: The Essential Guide to Nutrient Requirements.* National Academies Press, 2003.

272. Otto, G.P., M.Y. Wu, N. Kazgan, O.R. Anderson, and R.H. Kessin. 2003. Macroautophagy is required for multicellular development of the social amoeba *Dictyostelium discoideum*. *J Biol Chem* 278:17636–17645.

273. Oubidar, M., M. Boquillon, M.C. Bouvier, A. Beley, and J. Bralet. 1996. Effect of intracellular iron loading on lipid peroxidation of brain slices. *Free Radic Biol Med* 21, 763–769.

274. Paasche, G., D. Huster, and A. Reichenbach. 1998. The glutathione content of retinal Muller(glial) cells: the effects of aging and of application of free-radical scavengers. *Ophthalmic Res* 30:351–360.

275. Paddon-Jones, D., M. Sheffield-Moore, R.J. Urban, and

others. 2004a. Essential amino acid and carbohydrate supplementation ameliorates muscle protein loss during 28 days bedrest. *J Clin Endocrinol Metab* 89:4351–4358.

276. Paddon-Jones, D., M. Sheffield-Moore, X.J. Zhang, E. Volpi, S.E. Wolf, A. Aarsland, A.A. Ferrando, and R.R. Wolfe. 2004b. Amino acid ingestion improves muscle protein synthesis in the young and elderly. *Am J Physiol Endocrinol Metab* 286:E321–E328.

277. Paffenbarger Jr., R.S., J.B. Kampert, I.M. Lee, R.T. Hyde, and R.W. Leung. 1994. Changes in physical activity and other lifeway patterns influencing longevity. *Med Sci Sports Exerc* 26:857–865.

278. Pak, C.Y.C., K. Sakhaee, R.D. Peterson, J.R. Poindexter, W.H. Frawley. 2001. Biochemical profile of idiopathic uric acid nephrolithiasis. *Kidney International* 60:57–761.

279. Pak, C.Y.C, R.D. Peterson, and J. Poindexter. 2002. Prevention of spinal bone loss by potassium citrate in cases of calcium urolithiasis. *J Urol* 168:31–34.

280. Pallardó, F.V., M. Asensi, J. Garcia de l'Asuncion, V. Anton, A. Lloret, J. Sastre, and J. Vina. 1999. Late onset administration of oral antioxidants prevents age-related loss of motor coordination and brain mitochondrial DNA damage. *Free Radic Res* 29:617–623.

281. Panza, J.A., P.R. Casino, C.M. Kilcoyne, and A.A. Quyyumi. 1993. Role of endothelium-derived nitric oxide in the abnormal endothelium-dependent vascular relaxation of patients with essential hypertension. *Circulation* 87:1468–1474.

282. Parkes, T.L., A.J. Elia, D. Dickinson, A.J. Hilliker, J.P. Phillips, and G.L. Boulianne. 1998. Extension of *Drosophila* life span by overexpression of human SOD1 in motorneurons. *Nat Genet* 19:171–174.

283. Parks, J.H., L.A. Ruml, and C.Y.C. Pak. 1996. "Hypocitraturia." In Kidney Stones: Medical and Surgical Management, edited by F.L. Coe, M.J. Favus, C.Y.C Pak,

J.H. Parks, and G.M. Preminger, 905–920. Philadelphia: Lippincott-Raven, 1996.

284. Paolisso, G., S. Sgambato, A. Gambardella, G. Pizza, P. Tesauro, M. Varricchio, and F. D'Onofrio. 1992. Daily magnesium supplements improve glucose handling in elderly subjects. *Am J Clin Nutr* 55:1161–1167.

285. Phillips, S.M., K.D. Tipton, A. Aarsland, and others. 1997. Mixed muscle protein synthesis and breakdown after resistance exercise in humans. *Am J Physiol* 273:E99–1077.

286. Phuong-Chi Pham, T., T. Phuong-Mai Pham, V. Son Pham, J.M. Miller, and T. Phuong-Thu Pham. 2007. Hypomagnesemia in patients with type 2 diabetes. *Clin J Am Soc Nephrol* 2:366–373.

287. Pollock, M.L., G.A. Gaesser, J.D. Butcher, J-P Despres, R.K. Dishman, B.A. Franklin, and C.E. Garber. 1998. ACSM position stand: the recommended quantity and quality of exercise for developing and maintaining cardiorespiratory and muscular fitness, and flexibility in healthy adults. *Med Sci Sports and Exerc* 30:975–991.

288. Poon, H.F., V. Calabrese, M. Calvani, and D.A. Butterfield. 2006. Proteomics analyses of specific protein oxidation and protein expression in aged rat brain and its modulation by l-acetylcarnitine: insights into the mechanisms of action of this proposed therapeutic agent for CNS disorders associated with oxidative stress. *Antioxid Redox Signal* 8:381–394.

289. Pozefsky, T., P. Felig, J.C. Tobin, J.S. Soeldner, and G.F. Cahill Jr. 1969. Amino acids across tissues of the forearm in postabsorptive man. Effects of insulin at two dose levels. *J Clin Invest* 48:2273–2282.

290. Rabadjija, L., E.M. Brown, S.L. Swartz, C.J. Chen, and P. Goldhaber. 1990. H^+ stimulated release of prostaglandin E2 and cyclic adenosine 3',5'-monophosphoric acid and their relationship to bone resorption in neonatal mouse calvaria cultures. *Bone* 11:295–304.

291. Rafferty, K., K.M. Davies, and R.P. Heaney. 2005. Potassium intake and the calcium economy. *J Am Coll Nutr* 24:99–106.

292. Rantanen, T., T. Harris, S.G. Leveille, and others. 2000. Muscle strength and body mass index as long-term predictors for mobility in initially healthy men. *J Gerontol Med Sci* 55A:M168–M173.

293. Rapuri, P.B., J.C. Gallagher, and V. Haynatzka. 2003. Protein intake: effects on bone mineral density and the rate of bone loss in elderly women. *Am J Clin Nutr* 77:1517–1525.

294. Rasmussen, B.B., K.D. Tipton, S.L. Miller, S.E. Wolf, and R.R. Wolfe. 2000. An oral essential amino acid-carbohydrate supplement enhances muscle protein anabolism after resistance exercise. *J Appl Physiol* 88:386–392.

295. Rasmussen, B.B., R.R. Wolfe, and E. Volpi. 2002. Oral and intravenously administered amino acids produce similar effects on muscle protein synthesis in the elderly. *J Nutr Health Aging* 6:358–362.

296. Reggiori, F., and D.J. Klionsky. 2002. Autophagy in the eukaryotic cell. *Eukaryot Cell* 1:11–21.

297. Richwine, A.F., J.P. Godbout, B.M. Berg, J. Chem, J. Escobar, D.K. Millard, and R.W. Johnson. 2005. Improved psychomotor performance in aged mice fed diet high in antioxidants is associated with reduced ex *vivo* brain interleukin-6 production. *Brain Behav Immun* 19:512–520.

298. Ritcher, C. 1995. Oxidative damage to mitochondrial DNA and its relationship to ageing. *Int J Biochem Cell Biol* 27:647–653.

299. Rodriguez-Moran, M., and F. Guerrero-Romero. 2003. Oral magnesium supplementation improves insulin sensitivity and metabolic control in type 2 diabetic subjects. *Diabetes Care* 26:1147–1152.

300. Rosenblat, M., R. Coleman, and M. Avriam. 2002. Increased macrophage glutathione content reduces cell-mediated oxidation of LDL and atheroscelerosis in apolipoprotein E-deficient mice. *Artheroscelerosis* 163:17–28.

301. Rosendahl, E., N. Lindelöf, H. Littbrand, E. Yifter-Lindgren, L. Lundin-Olsson, L. Haglin, Y. Gustafson, and L. Nyberg. 2006. High-intensity functional exercise program and protein-enriched energy supplement for older persons dependent in activities of daily living: A randomized controlled trial. *Australian J Physio* 52:105–113.

302. Ross, R. 1999. Artheroscelerosis: an inflammation disease. *New Eng J Med* 340:115–126.

303. Russel, S.J., and C.R. Kahn. 2007. Endocrine regulation of ageing. Nature reviews. *Molecular Cell Biology* 8:681–691.

304. Sacheck, J.M., A. k Ohtsuka, C. McLary, and A.L. Goldberg. 2004. IGF-1 stimulates muscle growth by suppressing protein breakdown and expression of atrophy-related ubiquitin ligases, atrogin-1 and MuRF1. *Am J Physiol Endocrinol Metab* 287:E591–E601.

305. Sakhaee, K., N.M. Maalouf, S.A. Abrams, and C.Y.C Pak. 2005. Effects of potassium alkali and calcium supplementation on bone turnover in postmenopausal women. *J Clin Endocrinol & Metab* 90 (No. 6):3528–3533.

306. Salmeen, A., and D. Barford. 2005. Functions and mechanisms of redox regulation of cysteine-based phosphatases. *Antioxid Redox Signal* 7:560–577.

307. Sandri, M., C. Sandri, A. Gilbert, and others. 2004. FOXO transcription factors induce muscle atrophy. *Cell* 117:399–412.

308. Sasaki, T., M. Senda, S. Kim, S. Kojima, and A. Kubodera. 2001. Age-related changes of glutathione content, glucose transport and metabolism, and mitochondrial electron transfer function in mouse brain. *Nucl Med Biol* 28:25–31.

309. Sastre, J., M. Asensi, E. Gasco, F.V. Pallardo, J.A. Ferrero, T. Furukawa, and J. Vina. 1992. Exhaustive physical exercise causes oxidation of glutathione status in blood: Prevention by antioxidant administration. *Am J Physiol* 263:R992.

310. Sawka, M.N., S.N. Cheuvront, R. Carter 3rd. 2005. Human water needs. *Nutr Rev* 63:S30–S39.

311. Sayers, S.P. 2008. High-velocity power training in older adults. *Current Aging Science* 1:62–67.

312. Schmitt, T.L., A. Hotz-Wagenblatt, H. Klein, and W. Dröge. 2005. Interdependent regulation of insulin receptor kinase activity by ADP and hydrogen peroxide. *J Biol Chem* 280:3795–3801.

313. Scholze, A., C. Rinder, and J. Beige. 2004. Acetylcysteine reduces plasma homocysteine concentration and improves pulse pressure and endothelial function in patients with end-stage renal failure. *Circulation* 109:369–374.

314. Schutte, S.A., M.B. Zemel, and H.M. Linksweiler. 1980. Studies on the mechanism of protein-induced hypercalciuria in older men and women. *J Nutr* 110:305–315.

315. Scrofano, M.M., J. Jahngen-Hodge, T.R. Nowell, X. Gong, D.E. Smith, G. Peronne, G. Asmundsson, G. Dallal. B. Gindlesky, C.V. Mura, and A. Taylor. 1998. The effects of aging and calorie restriction on plasma nutrient levels in male and female Emory mice. *Mech Ageing Dev* 105:31–44.

316. Sebastian, A. 2005. Dietary protein content and the diet's net acid load: opposing effects on bone health. *Am J Clin Nutr* 82:921–922.

317. Sebastian, A., and R.C. Morris. 1994. Author's reply: mineral balance in postmenopausal women treated with potassium bicarbonate. *N Eng J Med* 331:1313.

318. Sebastien, A., S.T. Harris, J.H. Ottaway, K.M. Todd, and R.C. Morris Jr. 1994. Improved mineral balance and skeletal metabolism in postmenopausal women treated with potassium bicarbonate. *N Engl J Med* 330:1776–1781.

319. Sebastian, A., L. Frassetto, and R.C. Morris. 2005. Author's response: long-term persistenace of the urine calcium-lowering effect of potassium bicarbonate in postmenopausal women. *J Clin Endrocrin & Metab* 90(7):4417–4418.

320. Seeman, E., and P.D. Delmas. 2006. Bone quality: the material and structural basis of bone strength and fragility. *N Engl J Med* 354:2250–2261.

321. Sellmeyer, D., K.L. Stone, A. Sebastian, and S.R. Cummings. 2001. A high ratio of dietary animal to vegetable protein increases the rate of bone loss and the risk of fracture in postmenopausal women. *Am J Clin Nutr* 73:118–22.

322. Sellmeyer, D.E., M. Schloetter, and A. Sebastian. 2002. Potassium citrate prevents increased urine calcium excretion and bone resorption induced by a high sodium chloride diet. *J Clin Endocrinol Metab* 87:2008–2012.

323. Sen, C.K., T. Rankinen, S. Vaisanen, and R. Rauramaa. 1994. Oxidative stress after human exercise: Effect of N-acetylcysteine supplementation. *J Appl Physiol* 76:2570.

324. Shafiee, M.A., A.F. Charest, S. Cheema-Dhadli, D.N. Glick, O. Napolova, J. Roozbeh, E. Semenova, A. Sharman, and M.L. Halperin. 2005. Defining condition that lead to the retention of water: the importance of the arterial sodium concentration. *Kidney Int* 67 (2):613–621.

325. Shibata, H., H. Haga, M. Ueno, H. Nagai, S. Yasumura, and W. Koyano. 1991. Longitudinal changes of serum albumin in elderly people living in the community. *Age Aging* 20:417–420.

326. Shintani, T., and D.J. Klionsky. 2004. Autophagy in health and disease: a double-edged sword. *Science* 306:990–995.

327. Siani, A., P. Strazzullo, A. Giaco, D. Pacioni, E. Celentano, and M. Mancini. 1991. Increasing the dietary potassium intake reduces the need for antihypertensive medication. *Ann Intern Med.* 15:753–759.

328. Sigueira, I.R., C. Fochesatto, I. Lucena da Silva Torres, C. Dalmaz, and C.A. Netto. 2005. Aging affects oxidative state in hippocampus, hypothalamus and adrenal glands of Wistar rats. *Life Sciences* 78:271–278.

329. Siris, E.S., P.D. Miller, E. Barrett-Connor, K.G. Faulkner, L.E. Wehren, T.A. Abbott, M.L. Berger, A.C. Santora, and L.M. Sherwood LM. 2001. Identification and fracture outcomes of undiagnosed low bone mineral density

in postmenopausal women. Results from the National Osteoporosis Risk Assessment. *JAMA* 286:2815–2822.

330. Smaaland, R., K. Lote, and O. Sletvold. 1989. Circadian stage dependent variations in the DNA synthesis-phase and G2/M-phase of human bone marrow. *Proc Am Assoc Cancer Res* 30: 35.

331. Sohal, R.S., and B.H. Sohal. 1991. Hydrogen peroxide release by mitochondria increases during aging. *Mech Ageing Dev* 57:187–202.

332. Sohal, R., and R. Weindruch. 1996. Oxidative stress, caloric restriction, and aging. *Science* 273:59–67.

333. Sohal, R., E. Weenberg-Kirch, K. Jaiswal, L.K. Kwong, and M.J. Forster. 1999. Effect of age and caloric restriction on bleomycin-chelatable and non-heme iron in different tissues of C57BL/6 mice. *Free Radic Biol Med* 27:287–293.

334. Sohal, R.S., R.J. Mockett, and W.C Orr. 2002. Mechanisms of ageing: an appraisal of the oxidative stress hypothesis. *Free Radic Biol Med* 33:575–586.

335. Solomon, A., and A. Goldberg. 1996. Importance of the ATP-ubiquitin-proteasome pathway in the degradation of soluble and myofibrillar proteins in rabbit muscle extracts. *J Biol Chem* 271:26690–26697.

336. Sprague, S.M., N.S. Krieger, and D.A. Bushinsky. 1994. Greater inhibition of in vitro bone mineralization with metabolic than respiratory acidosis. *Kidney Int* 46:1199–1209.

337. Standing Committee on the Scientific Evaluation of Dietary Reference Intakes. Dietary Reference Intakes for Calcium, Phosphorus, Magnesium, Vitamin D, and Fluoride. Washington DC: National Academy Press, 1997.

338. Stipanuk, M.H., R.M. Coloso, R.A. Garcia, and M.F. Banks. 1992. Cysteine concentration regulates cysteine metabolism to glutathione, sulfate and taurine in rat hepatocytes. *J Nutr* 122(3):420–427.

339. Stitt, T.N., D. Drujan, B.A. Clarke, and others. 2004. The

IGF-1/P13K/Akt pathway prevents expression of muscle atrophy-induced ubiquitin ligases by inhibiting FOXO transcription factors. *Mol Cell* 14:395–403.

340. Stöckler, S., U. Holzbach, F. Hanefeld, I. Marquardt, G. Helms, M. Requart, W. Hänicke, and J. Frahm. 1994. Creatine deficiency in the brain: a new treatable inborn error of metabolism. *Pediatr Res* 36: 409–413.

341. Stöckler-Ipsiroglu, S. 1997. Creatine deficiency syndromes: a new perspective on metabolic disorders and a diagnostic challenge. *J Pediatr* 131:510–511.

342. Stupina, A., A. Terman, T. Kvitmitskaia-Ryzhova, N.A. Mezhiborkaia, and V.A. Zherebitskii. 1994. The age-related characteristics of autophagocytosis in different tissues of laboratory animals. *Tsitologiia Genetika* 28:15–20.

343. Swanberg, E., A.C. Moller-Loswick, D.E. Matthews, U. Korner, M. Andersson, and K. Lundholm. 1999. The role of glucose, long-chain triglycerides and amino acids for promotion of amino acid balance across peripheral tissues in man. *Clin Physiol* 19:311–320.

344. Tallóczy, Z., W. Jiang, H.W. Virgin IV, D.A. Leib, D. Scheuner, R.J. Kaufman, E-L Eskelinen, and B. Levine. 2002. Regulation of starvation- and virus-induced autophagy by the eIF2α kinase signaling pathway. *Proc Natl Acad Sci* 99:190–195.

345. Taub, J., J.F. Lau, C. Ma, J.H. Hahn, R. Hoque, J. Rothblatt, and M. Chalfie. 1999. A cytosolic catalase is needed to extend adult life span in *C. elegans daf-C* and *elk-1 mutants*. *Nature* 399:162–166.

346. Tepel, M., M. Van Der Giet, and M. Statz. 2003. The Antioxidant acetylcysteine reduces cardiovascular events in patients with end-stage renal failure: A randomized, controlled trial. *Circulation* 107:992–995.

347. Terman, A. 1995. The effect of age on formation an elimination of autophagic vacuoles in mouse hepatocyte. *Gerontology* 41:319–325.

348. Terman, A. H. Dalen, J.W. Eaton, J. Neuzil, and U.T. Brunk. 2003. Mitochondrial recycling and aging of cardiac myocytes: the role of autophagocytosis. *Exp Gerontol* 38:863–876.

349. Thomas, D.R. 2007. Loss of skeletal muscle mass in aging: examining the relationship of starvation, sarcopenia and cachexia. *Clin Nutr* 26:389–399.

350. Tipton, K.D, A.A. Ferrando, S.M. Phillips, D. Doyle Jr., and R.R. Wolfe. 1999. Postexercise net protein synthesis in human muscle from orally administered amino acids. *Am J Physiol* 276:E628–634.

351. Tipton, K.D., B.B. Rasmussen, S.L. Miller, S.E. Wolf, S.K. Owens-Stovall, B.E. Petrini, and R.R. Wolfe. 2001. Timing of amino acid-carbohydrate ingestion alters anabolic response of muscle to resistance exercise. *Am J Physiol Endocrinol Metab* 281:E197–E206.

352. Tipton, K.D., E. Borsheim, S.E. Wolf, A.P. Sanford, and R.R. Wolfe. 2003. Acute response of net muscle protein balance reflects 24-h balance after exercise and amino acid ingestion. *Am J Physiol Endocrinol Metab* 284:E76–E89.

353. Tipton, K.D., T.A. Elliott, M.G. Cree, S.E. Wolf, A.P. Sanford, and R.R. Wolfe. 2004. Ingestion of casein and whey proteins result in muscle anabolism after resistance exercise. *Med Sci Sports Exerc* 2073–2081.

354. Tiselius, H.G. 2001. Possibilities for preventing recurrent calcium stone formation: principles for the metabolic evaluation of patients with calcium stone disease. *BJU International* 88:158–168.

355. Touyz, R.M. 2004. Reactive oxygen species, vascular oxidative stress, and redox signaling in hypertension: what is the clinical significance? *Hypertension* 44:248–252.

356. Traverso, N., S. Patriarca, E. Balbis, A.L. Furfaro, D. Cottalasso, M.A. Pronzato, P. Carlier, F. Botta, U.M. Marinari, and L. Fontana. 2003. Anti malondialdehyde-adduct immunological response as a possible marker of successful aging. *Exp Gerontol* 38:1129–1135.

357. Tremblay, F., M. Krebs, L. Dombrowski, A. Brehm, E. Bernroider, E. Roth, P. Nowotny, W. Waldhausl, A. Marette, and M. Roden. 2005. Overactivation of S6 kinase 1 as a cause of human insulin resistance during increased amino acid availability. *Diabetes* 54:2674–2684.

358. Tsukada, M., and Y. Ohsumi. 1993. Isolation and characterization of autophagy-defective mutants of *Saccharomyces cerevisiae*. *FEBS Lett* 333:169–174.

359. Tucker, K.L., M.T. Hannan, H. Chen, L.A. Cupples, P.W.F. Wilson, and D.P. Kiel. 1999. Potassium, magnesium, and fruit and vegetable intakes are associated with greater bone mineral density in elderly men and women. *Am J Clin Nutr* 69:727–736.

360. Ushmorov, A., V. Hack, and W. Dröge. 1999. Differential reconstitution of mitochondrial respiratory chain activity and plasma redox state by cysteine and ornthine in a model of cancer cachexia. *Cancer Res* 59:3527–3534.

361. Van der Loo, B., M. Bachschmid, V. Spitzer, L. Brey, V. Ullrich, and T.F. Lüscher. 2003. Decreased plasma and tissue levels of vitamin C in a rat model of aging: implications for antioxidative defense. *Biochem Biophys Res Commun* 303:483–487.

362. Van Remmen, H., Y. Ikeno, M. Hamilton, M. Pahlavani, N. Wolf, S.R. Thorpe, N.L. Alderson, J.W. Baynes, C.J. Epstein, T-T Huang, J. Nelson, R. Strong, and A. Richardson. 2003. Lifelong reduction in MnSOD activity results in increased DNA damage and higher incidence of cancer but does not accelerate aging. *Physiol Geonomics* 16:29–37.

363. Vassilakopoulos, T., M-H Karatza, P. Katsaounou, A. Kollintza, S. Zakynthinos, and C. Roussos. 2003. Antioxidants attenuate the plasma cytokine response to exercise in humans. *J Appl Physiol* 94:1025–1032.

364. Vijg, J., and J. Campisi. 2008. Puzzles, promises and a cure for ageing. *Nature* 454:1065–1071.

365. Volpi, E., A.A. Ferrando, C.W. Yeckel, K.D. Tipton,

and R.R. Wolfe. 1998. Exogenous amino acids stimulate net muscle protein synthesis in the elderly. *J Clin Invest* 101:2000–2007.

366. Volpi, E., B. Mittendorfer, S.E. Wolf, and R.R. Wolfe. 1999. Oral amino acids stimulate muscle protein anabolism in the elderly despite higher first-pass splanchnic extraction. *Am J Physiol* 277:E513–520.

367. Volpi, E., H. Kobayashi, M. Sheffield-Moore, B. Mittendorfer, and R.R. Wolfe. 2003. Essential amino acids are primarily responsible for the amino acid stimulation of muscle protein anabolism in healthy elderly adults. *Am J Clin Nutr* 78:250–258.

368. Volpi, S.L. 2008. Magnesium, the metabolic syndrome, insulin resistance, and type 2 diabetes mellitus. *Crit Rev Food Sci Nutr* 48:293–300.

369. Walker, R.M., and H. Linkswiler. 1972. Calcium retention in the adult human male as affected by protein intake. *J Nutr* 102:1297–1302.

370. Wang, C.W., and D.J. Klionsky. 2003. The molecular mechanism of autophagy. *Mol Med* 9:65–76.

371. Weger, W., P. Kotanko, M. Weger, H. Deutschmann, and F. Skrabal. 2000. Prevalence and characterization of renal tubular acidosis in patients with osteopenia and osteoporosis and in nonporotic controls. *Nephrol Dial Transplant* 15:975–980.

372. Weindruch, R., and R.L. Walford. *The Retardation Of Aging And Disease By Dietary Restriction.* Springfield, Ill.: Charles C. Thomas, 1988.

373. Weindruch, R., and R.L. Walford. 1997. Caloric intake and aging. *N Engl J Med* 337, 986–994.

374. Welle, S. *Human Protein Metabolism.* New York: Springer, 1999.

375. Welle, S., and C.A. Thornton. 1998. High-protein meals do not enhance myofibrillar synthesis after resistance exercise in

62- to 75 yr-old men and women. *Am J Physiol* 274:E677–683.

376. Welle, S., C. Thornton, R. Jozefowicz, and M. Statt. 1993. Myofibrillar protein synthesis in young and old men. *Am J Physiol* 264:E693–698.

377. Wessells, R.J., E. Fitzgerald, J.R. Cypser, Tatar, and R. Bodmer. 2004. Insulin regulation of heart function in aging fruit flies. *Nat Genet* 36:1275–1281.

378. Wolfe, R.R. 2006. The underappreciated role of muscle in health and disease. *Am J Clin Nutr* 84:475–482.

379. Woo, J. 2000. Relationships among diet, physical activity and other lifestyle factors and debilitating diseases in the elderly. *Eur J Clin Nutr* 54 (Suppl 3):143–147.

380. Wood, R.J. 1994. Mineral balance in postmenopausal women treated with potassium bicarbonate. *N Eng J Med* 331:1312–1313.

381. Yarasheski, K.E., J.J. Zachwieja, and D.M. Bier. 1993. Acute effects of resistance exercise on muscle protein synthesis rate in young and elderly men and women. *Am J Physiol* 265:E210–214.

382. Yi, J., and X.M. Tang. 1995. Functional implication of autophagy in steroid-secreting cells of the rat. *Anatomic Rec* 242:137–146.

383. Yokota, S., M. Himeno, J. Roth, D. Brada, and K. Kato. 1993. Formation of autophagosomes during degradation of excess peroxisomes induced by di-(2-ethylhexyl)phthalate treatment. II. Immunocytochemical analysis of early and late autophagosomes. *Eur J Cell Biol* 62:372–383.

384. Yoon, J.C., P. Puigserver, G. Chen, J. Donovan, Z. Wu, J. Rhee, G. Adelmant, J. Stafford, C.R. Kahn, D.K. Granner, C.B. Newgard, and B. Spiegelman. 2001. Control of hepatic gluconeogenesis through the transcriptional coactivator PGC-1. *Nature* 413:131–138.

385. Young, V.R. 1990. Amino acids and proteins in relation to the nutrition of elderly people. *Age Ageing* 19:S10–S24.

386. Zhao, J., J.J. Brault, A. Schild, P. Cao, M. Sandri, S. Schiaffino, S.H. Lecker, and A.L. Goldberg. 2007. FoxO3 coordinately activates protein degradation by the autophagic/lysosomal and proteasomal pathways in atrophying muscle cells. *Cell Metabolism* 6:472–483.

387. Zheng, J., R. Mutcherson II, and S.L. Helfand. 2005. Calorie restriction delays lipid oxidative damage in *Drosophila melanogaster*. *Aging Cell* 4:209–216.

388. Zhu, Y., P.M. Carvey, and Z. Ling. 2006. Age-related changes in glutathione and glutathione-related enzymes in rat brain. *Brain Res* 1090:35–44.

389. Ziegenfuss, T.N., M. Rogers, L. Lowery, N. Mullins, R. Mendel, J. Antonio, and P. Lemon. 2002. Effect of creatine loading on anaerobic performance and skeletal muscle volume in NCAA Division I athletes. *Nutrition* 18:398–402.

Index

Addendum One: Practical Guidelines

Limits of a Rigid Guideline

A rigid guideline can never substitute for a deeper understanding of the content and implications of the previous chapters. Incorporating these principles into ones life is like an art that takes months or years to perfect. Also, the design of a rigid guideline cannot fully rely on published scientific studies but is largely based on personal experience, common sense and anecdotal observations. Parameters such as doses or timing have not been systematically investigated in most of the scientific studies available.

Certain disadvantages of the interventions described in this book could possibly be minimized by repeatedly measuring various physical, biochemical, and metabolic parameters, but these are usually not available to the non-specialist. In view of these challenges, these interventions have been integrated here into one flexible program that is somewhat simplistic but can be followed blindly. Rapamycin has not been included in this program as long as there are no safety data from clinical trials available.

Program Schedule One: The Cysteine Supplementation Mode

The schedule in figure 13 may be viewed as a standard schedule for cysteine supplementation that may be modified according to the individual needs. It is recommended to consume approximately 15 to 60 grams of a cysteine-rich whey protein supplement per day corresponding to 0.4 to 1.6 grams cysteine depending on the individual body weight and the intensity of the physical exercise activity. If a portion of 10 to 50 grams of this whey protein is consumed immediately before or after a bout of physical exercise, this schedule strongly supports not only the synthesis of glutathione, but also the synthesis of skeletal muscle proteins needed to ameliorate the age-related loss of muscle mass and muscle function. The term supplement means that whey protein is consumed in addition to other types of proteins contained in the normal diet.

Program Schedule Two: The Creatine Supplementation Mode

Creatine is being used to avoid or reverse the undesirable change in plasma cystine concentration and redox state after prolonged consumption of cysteine supplements. It is recommended to follow the schedule one (cysteine supplementation without creatine) only for two or three days and to switch subsequently to the use of cysteine in combination with creatine. Specifically, 0.04 grams of creatine may be added to each gram of whey protein. As this amount of creatine is typically contained in about 8 grams of beef, creatine supplementation is not needed by persons who happen to consume large amounts of meat. Diabetic patients may face additional challenges as discussed in chapter three.

The main disadvantage of this procedure is that the non-specialist cannot monitor and adequately adjust the moderate reduction in *basal* insulin signaling activity in the fasted state which would be expected to reverse the age-related decline in autophagy. It is therefore recommended to switch after a few days to program schedule three (calorie restriction) as a kind of reset mode.

Program Schedule Three: Calorie Restriction as a Reset Mode

Calorie restriction is usually not enjoyable. But with the awareness of the important benefits one is in the position to chose the number of calories per day responsibly. If the blood pressure decreases and one starts feeling cold at night one is on the right track. One should keep in mind that rigorous restriction requires special attention to the daily essentials such as minerals, vitamins and the protein supply. A deficiency in dietary protein may cause fatigue, muscle pain and loss of hair quality. Before applying rigorous calorie restriction, one may want to talk to a medical professional. It is recommended to practice calorie restriction only for short periods of one or a few days before *gradually* increasing again the tissue creatine pools by switching back to schedule two as a reconstructive mode and then eventually to schedule one (Cysteine Supplementation) to restart the program. By limiting calorie restriction to a few days at a time with intermittent periods of vigorous reconstruction of muscle mass and function, one may be able to get important benefits while minimizing the negative trade-offs. If the blood pressure should increase during schedule one, one may switch directly to schedule two: the blood pressure is likely to decrease again after one or two days.

The schedules one and three place the major emphasis on "waste-removal" and related biological activities. This process is most important for life span extension (see previous chapters) but the auto-cannibalism will eventually lead to some degree of muscle weakness and fatigue. At this point one may switch to schedule two which places major emphasis on skeletal muscle protein synthesis at the expense of "waste-removal" and related functions. As these latter functions are generally "invisible" and typically happen during the night, schedule two is perceived as the most comfortable schedule. It should never be forgotten, however, that the most important processes for life span extension are not the maintenance of muscle mass and muscle function but rather the processes of "waste-removal" and related activities.

Water-assisted Autophagy and Supplementation of Magnesium and Citric Acid Salts

Throughout the program one may use *water-assisted autophagy* as a supporting procedure to enhance autophagy and amino acid homeostasis. Also, attention shoul be given to adequate supplements of magnesium and citric acid salts to maintain a good acid-base balance. The urine pH should be adjusted to a value of approximately 6.5 to 6,8 (see chapter 7). It is conceivable that low doses of rapamycin supplements during the night (before sleeping) may also become popular in the future when clinical data on safety become available. Living by the principles described here will eventually be developed into an art.

Addendum Two:
Comment on the Rapamycin Study and the IT Program

The report by Harrison and colleagues on the effect of rapamycin in old mice (Nature **460**, 393;2009) suggests that in the not so distant future humans will be able to live substantially longer than 120 years with good health and quality of life. The authors were fair enough to point out, however, that the mammalian target of rapamycin (mTOR) is not only a devil that shortens life span but also an important signaling element with positive functions in the metabolic (mostly synthetic) response to food intake. As mTOR is a part of the insulin signaling pathway, life span extension by rapamycin is reminiscent of the life span extension seen in various animal mutants with an impairment in autologoues of the insulin receptor and its signaling cascade. Several studies in mutants of C.elegans have indicated that autophagy and FOXO transcription factor activity are required for life span extension. As these functions are typically suppressed by this signaling pathway as well as by amino acids through TOR they are almost inactive after food intake and most active in the starved condition. Aging is generally associated with a decrease in autophagic activity and an accumulation of "cellular waste". Silencing of mTOR is therefore most critically required in the starved condition (that is in humans during the night) and not after food intake. There is reason to believe that the encapsulation of the drug as used in the study of Harrison and colleagues might have been important for its success by serving as a kind of "slow-release" device. This might have helped to exert at least some effect on the postabsorptive (that is the starved) period and a lesser effect on rapamycin-dependent synthetic processes in the period immediately after food intake. In view of these arguments and the mechanisms described in this book, the US National Institute on Aging's Intervention Testing Program (ITP) may be expected to benefit if the candidate compounds were generally tested in slow-release formulations with a twelve hours delay in delivery.

About the Author

Wulf Dröge studied chemistry and biochemistry at the University of Freiburg, Germany, and served for three years as a postdoctoral research fellow at Harvard University and for four years as a scientific member at the Basel Institute for Immunology in Switzerland. From 1976 to 2005, he was head of a department at the National Cancer Research Center of Germany (Deutsches Krebsforschungszentrum) in Heidelberg and professor of immunology and cell biology at the University of Heidelberg. He is presently living in Montreal, Canada. He is a member of several scientific societies. His main research areas include redox regulation, oxidative stress, aging, and the mechanisms of disease-related wasting. This book has been inspired by many years of research in his own laboratory.